HEALTH CARE FOR AN AGING SOCIETY

HEALTH CARE FOR AN AGING SOCIETY
Cost-Conscious Community Care and Self-Care Approaches

David Haber
School of Medicine, Creighton University

Routledge
Taylor & Francis Group
NEW YORK AND LONDON

HEALTH CARE FOR AN AGING SOCIETY: Cost-Conscious Community Care and Self-Care Approaches

This edition by Routledge:

Routledge
Taylor and Francis Group
711 Third Avenue,
New York, NY 10017

Routledge
Taylor and Francis Group
2 Park Square, Milton Park, Abingdon,
Oxfordshire OX14 4RN

First issued in hardback 2017

Routledge is an imprint of the Taylor and Francis Group, an informa business

Cover design by Debra Eubanks Riffe.

Library of Congress Cataloging-in-Publication Data

Haber, David
Health care for aging society: cost-conscious community care and self-care approaches / David Haber.
p. cm. — (Series in death education, aging, and health care)
Bibliography: p.
Includes index.

1. Medical care, Cost of—United States. 2. Medical policy—United States. 3. Aged—United States—Long term care. 4. Aged—Medical care—United States. I. Title. II. Series.
[DNLM: 1. Community Health Services—economics. 2. Cost Control. 3. Health Services for the Aged—economics. 4. Long Term Care—economics. 5. Self care—economics. WT 30 H114h]
RA410.53.H33 1989
338.4'73621'989700973—dc 19
DNLM/DLC
for Library of Congress 88-38304
CIP

ISBN 13: 978-1-138-18014-7 (hbk)
ISBN 13: 978-1-56032-227-6 (pbk)
ISSN 0275-3510

To Benjamin and Audrey

CONTENTS

III
COST-CONSCIOUS SELF-CARE APPROACHES

APPENDIXES

PREFACE

In the era of cost containment the challenge of rising medical costs continues to be difficult. In an aging society, however, the challenge broadens to include health care and social support at home and in the community. The major premise of this book is that cost-conscious community care and self-care will become increasingly important as the era of cost containment intensifies.

During the first half of the 1980s, health care cost containment strategies targeted the major arenas of cost escalation, the acute care and institutional sectors. While this battle continues to rage, another has begun in long-term care. An aging society must contend with an increased number of persons with chronic care conditions and a demand for more long-term care services at home and in the community.

Typically these services fall outside the traditional medical care model and include such activities as home health care, home care, respite care, community volunteer networks, lay education, professional geriatric education, health promotion, prevention, family caregiving, self-help groups, and social support. Advocacy for additional long-term care services is often justified on the basis of cost reductions in the acute care and institutional sectors. Much of the evidence suggests, however, that additional long-term care services are not necessarily cost-effective alternatives, but additional needed services.

No matter which way the public/private seesaw rises in terms of financial responsibility for these additional services, the bottom line is that long-term care depends on people. The next decade will test our capacity to support the family, strengthen the community, enhance the congregation, engage the corporation, educate the professional, and empower the individual.

Part One describes the era of cost containment. After decades of rapid health care cost escalation in the acute care and institutional sectors, a wide variety of cost containment practices have been implemented recently. As the era of cost containment intensifies, the additional challenge of meeting the demand for long-term care at home and in the community is upon us.

Chapter 1 begins with a brief summary of 4 decades of rising medical expenditures. To meet the challenge of rising costs, the fee-for-service, retrospective reimbursement system has been quickly giving way to prospective payment systems or managed care. DRGs, HMOs, PPOs, regulatory restructuring, competition, and other cost containment strategies have become familiar refrains not only to policymakers and practitioners but to the lay public as well.

Chapters 2 and 3 point out that long-term care is a separate, but related, arena to the acute care and institutional issues that dominated the early 1980s. In the late 1980s we are coming to realize that society must provide additional services to cope with chronic care conditions and that these home- and community-based services will not be financed through cost reductions in the acute or institutional care sectors.

More specifically, Chapter 2 discusses the implications of an aging society, a society in which older persons are the most rapidly aging segment of the population and where the caregiving burden falls disproportionately on the backs of women. While the American Association of Retired Persons and other organizations have done much to raise public awareness during the past few years the majority of Americans do not acknowledge their long-term care vulnerabilities. A variety of long-term care myths are examined, and what remains is the need for more support for older persons and their families at home and in the community.

Chapter 3 examines long-term care services, both comprehensive and piecemeal approaches. National and regional research studies report that community-based alternatives do not reduce overall health care costs. On the other hand, much can be done to alleviate the burdens of long-term care in an aging society. The present shotgun approach to implementing and examining comprehensive and piecemeal strategies, public and private reimbursement systems, and institutional and community-based services is understandable in light of the brief era of cost containment and a short history of program development.

Part Two examines a wide range of cost-conscious community care options, from the ubiquitous family caregiver and volunteer network to the promise that congregations and corporations have for mobilizing additional long-term care resources. The provision of cost-conscious community care requires the training of caregiving professionals and laypersons alike.

Chapter 4 reinforces the idea that the heart of the health care system for an aging society is home care and family caregiving. Due to demographical, physiological, economical, and social factors, support in the home will be harder to come by. A review of the many interesting variations of family caregiving in today's society may offer insight into the unique ways that families cope with limited resources. In addition, neighbors and volunteers can be as important as family for maintaining independence in the home.

Chapter 5 focuses on two largely untapped resources in an aging society. While older persons constitute the largest age group in organized religion, religious leaders tend not to have gerontological training. There is great potential to mobilize the energy of congregational members toward the problems of aging and family caregiving.

A tremendous surge of wellness activities at the work site has occurred over the past decade. Much of this effort is directed toward those already committed to physical fitness. A small but growing interest in the wellness of the older worker, however, has begun to appear as well. One topic of particular interest, especially to women, is the dual responsibility of working outside the home and caring for an older relative, which currently affects 25% of the work force. Work-site elder care programs are emerging to meet these often conflicting responsibilities.

Chapter 6 documents the need that the vast majority of health care professionals have for basic geriatric knowledge. Moreover, as people grow older, their health needs become more complex and interdependent, and the 200 different types of health care personnel providing services to the elderly must learn to collaborate with each other as well. Professionals, in addition, need to learn how to work with the informal caregiving network and the community resource persons that older persons depend on for support with their chronic care problems. The national network of geriatric education centers and the Creighton Center for Healthy Aging are two responses to the need for geriatric education among and between health care professionals and health consumers.

Part Three focuses on the cost-conscious self-care approaches of health promotion and self-help groups. While these strategies emphasize individual empowerment, they are viewed in the context of professional-layperson collaboration and a stronger advocacy role in both the public and private arenas.

The ideal health care system for an aging society is one that keeps people healthy. Chapter 7 focuses on the three most popular forms of health promotion and aging: exercise, nutrition, and stress management. In addition, an increasing number of comprehensive wellness and self-care programs target older people.

Chapter 8 highlights the self-help movement with its accent on empowerment, accessibility, and personal experience. By almost any measure of growth, the self-help movement is a phenomenon to be reckoned with. Some of the challenges of the upcoming decade are to involve more older persons and their family caregivers, to enhance the ability to reach out to lower economic sectors of society, and to link these peer-led groups more effectively with health care professionals.

The concluding chapter summarizes the book's content. Rising health care costs and a growing demand for home- and community-based long-term care services in an era of limited resources challenge both service providers and policymakers to develop new programs that are responsive to an aging society. These programs must be holistic and interdisciplinary, with an accent on the education of laypersons and professionals, as well as the interaction between them. Also, while there will always be a need for government leadership and support, we must strengthen the wellness and caregiving capacities of congregations, corporations, and self-help groups.

The resource appendixes provide a comprehensive listing of national aging resource organizations. They also cover several areas often overlooked by other resource directories that have been compiled to serve the needs of older persons and caregivers. Appendix C, in addition, includes a health promotion and aging bibliography.

David Haber

ACKNOWLEDGMENTS

I want to thank Benjamin and Audrey for being so lovable. I will always strive to be the father that you two deserve. I want to thank Charles Monasee, executive director of the Health Future Foundation, and Richard O'Brien, MD, vice-president of Creighton University's Schools of Health Sciences, for supporting the unique vision called the Creighton Center for Healthy Aging.

I

ERA OF COST CONTAINMENT

1

CHALLENGE OF RISING MEDICAL COSTS

An examination of American health care over the past few decades reveals skyrocketing cost escalation due to the growth in the number of hospitals and nursing homes and the intensive medical services and extensive custodial services associated with these institutions. A summary of this cost escalation and the advent of the cost containment era is important for three reasons. First, it helps us understand why it is so difficult to generate public resources for a long-term care system, despite the hoards of elders with chronic care needs who will be approaching this system over the upcoming decades. Second, it reminds us that no matter how urgently we need long-term health care and social services we are going to have to depend a great deal on no-cost and low-cost services. Third, additional public monies allocated to long-term care alternatives may have to be justified on cost-effective grounds; that is, additional funds allocated to long-term care alternatives will result in a comparable reduction in expenditures in the acute care and institutional sectors.

COST ESCALATION

The problem of escalating health care costs began at the conclusion of World War II, when tremendous shortages in health care manpower and hospital bed capacity were revealed (McNerney, 1983). These shortages led to substantial federally supported programs to increase enrollment in medical schools. Graduate and postgraduate training programs grew steadily from the 1950s through the 1970s. In addition, the military medical research budget after World War II was transferred to and institutionalized through the National Institutes of Health. By the late 1970s, 90% of biomedical research was funded by the federal government (Califano, 1986).

The 1946 Hill-Burton Act made grants and loans available for building and equipping hospitals and other health care facilities. Almost two thirds of all American hospitals were built or modernized through this program. Throughout the 1950s and 1960s this act was vital for expanding the capacity of health care facilities to meet the growing health care demands of Americans. While it was successful in expanding hospital bed capacity, many analysts held this program partly responsible for the overbuilding of hospitals and the resulting excess bed capacity (Butler, 1975). By 1986 excess hospital beds totaled 34% of existing supply. Analysts estimate that unfilled beds generate more than one half of the costs of their filled counterparts due to the pressure to expand staff and medical services (Juster & Lanning, 1982). These costs were not recouped because the beds remained empty. Had the cost containment era arrived earlier, the elimination of excess beds would have saved many billions of dollars over the past 2 decades (Califano, 1986).

Escalating health care costs were not merely a consequence of increased medical training, research, and hospital beds. The numbers and the costs of health care procedures and the use of complex machinery rose dramatically as well. Medical breakthroughs in the 1960s and 1970s extended to CAT scanners, dialysis, surgical bypasses, drug therapies, pacemakers, total hip replacements, and an endless variety of clinical laboratory tests (Banta et al., 1983; Berki, 1983). The next generation of applied health care technology, such as magnetic resonance scanners and positive emission tomographers, has been introduced to hospitals in the 1980s, and it promises to be equally impressive in terms of both achievement and expenditure. Therefore, many of the cost containment practices during this period have been consequences of circumstance rather than public policy that provides cost containment guidelines. An example of this is organ transplantation. Kidney and pancreas transplants in the 1980s (costing up to $50,000 each in 1984) and heart and liver transplants (costing up to $35,000) have been limited primarily by the availability of organs, not by public policy on health care cost containment.

Another cost-escalating factor has been a reliance on surgical interventions. In comparison to patients in other nations, Americans are the recipients of more surgical procedures despite the fact that this higher incidence of surgery does not correlate with improved medical outcomes (McClure, 1983). As these costly services and procedures multiplied, so has the ratio of employees per hospital bed, from approximately two to three per bed during the 1970s (Schoen et al., 1983) to four per bed in the 1980s (Califano, 1986). This is a much higher ratio than exists in European countries where sophisticated health care systems are also in place.

Over the past few decades health care has become costly because of a wide variety of factors: the expanding supply of physicians and other health care specialists to serve the increasing number of hospital and nursing home beds; the application of technological advances; general inflation and the even more rapid health inflation in the economy; hospital-based diagnostic and surgical technologies and excessive hospital stays; greater intensity of medical care provided, including the overspecialization of physicians; increased cost of medical malpractice insurance and excessive medical tests; subsidized inefficiency and profiteering in the nursing home industry; tax subsidies to employees and tax deductions to employer health care programs; and the aging of Americans, who incur more chronic or catastrophic conditions in later life.

Perhaps the most influential factor of all, however, has been the third-party, fee-for-service, retrospective payment system. This system encourages high medical care utilization and expensive treatment modalities and discourages cost containment practices. In 1983 almost three fourths of personal health expenditures were paid through third-party payments (U.S. Senate Special Committee on Aging, 1985). *Third-party payments,* in brief, are expenditures that are made by government agencies or insurance companies to health care providers. Thus, the painful link between goods and services being consumed and the consumer's wallet has been, for the most part, severed.

What was not severed was the link between third-party payers and health care providers. Prior to 1981 health care providers constituted over half of the membership on the board of directors at Blue Cross/Blue Shield, the nation's largest insurance intermediary. Thus, physicians and hospital administrators were in the position of approving payments for whatever their colleagues were charging (Califano, 1986). After much pressure new policies requiring nonprovider board members were approved in 1982 by Blue Cross/Blue Shield.

Fee for service simply means more services will generate more fees. The provider who practices a conservative style of medical care is penalized, while the provider who uses extensive services, acute care hospitals, and expensive technology is rewarded. Merely limiting hospital stays and visits to the physician is not effective in limiting the fee-for-service system. As the U.S. Senate Special Committee on Aging (1985) reports, hospital stays and visits to the physician by the elderly increased a modest 26% during the 1970s, but physicians' bills for service increased 220%. Up until recently the only method to contain the climbing costs of physician services was to set predetermined fees for specific services as in health maintenance organizations, thereby making physicians financially responsible for living within a budget. In the past few years another option has been proposed, fee for outcome (Kane et al., 1983), where payment is made only for those services that attain achievable medical goals.

Finally the *retrospective* nature of the fee-for-service system has undermined the capacity of government or private health care organizations and physicians to plan ahead or to foster restraint on the use of medical care. In the absence of prospectively determined budgets, the only option has been a post hoc strategy to generate revenues.

SHIFTING TO PROSPECTIVE PAYMENT SYSTEMS

It was not until the mid 1970s that the problems of escalating health care costs and expanding hospital beds and manpower were addressed. The 1974 National Health Planning and Resources Development Act, for instance, shifted federal attention from constructing additional hospitals to modernizing existing facilities, improving efficiency of care, and containing capital costs (McNerney, 1983). The 1976 Health Professions Act also shifted the focus from expanding the ranks of health care personnel to redistributing the existing manpower to underserved areas.

Perhaps the most dramatic shift of all began in the late 1970s and early 1980s, when the fee-for-service, retrospective reimbursement system was being replaced by prospective payment systems at the corporate, state, and federal levels. After several years of experimentation with techniques for monitoring and controlling health care costs, prepayments became the major alternative to the generous reimbursement policies of the past decades. *Prospective payment system* refers to a set of rules to pay providers in advance instead of after the fact. This system helps set limits on costs and establish plans to generate necessary and predictable revenue levels. Many prepayment systems allow providers to earn profits if actual costs are below approved rates.

It is important to note at the onset, however, that a prospective payment system can be virtually indistinguishable from retrospective reimbursements. A modified prospective system, for instance, can allow liberal adjustments or exceptions for costs incurred after the fact. Thus, modified systems can escalate costs on a par with cost-based retrospective systems (Tynan et al., 1981).

In general, preliminary studies report that prospective payment systems are associated with lower expenditures (Waldo & Lazenby, 1984). These cost savings have prompted an increasing number of states to terminate their retrospective payment systems in nursing homes (Waldo & Lazenby, 1984). Sloan (1983) reports that prospective payment systems in hospitals have in some instances prompted a yearly cost inflation savings of about 3% to 4% after 3 years of operation, provided the rate setting is mandatory rather than voluntary. Sloan and others conclude that prospective payment systems are most likely to be effective when the level of payment strikes a balance—if the rate setting is too high per individual or diagnosis, it removes the incentive for cost efficiency; if too low, quality and access will be compromised (Ochsner, 1983; Sloan, 1983).

While prospective payment systems in general hold much promise, they are not panaceas and can produce undesirable and unintended outcomes. Preliminary studies show the major concerns to be lower quality care, limited access for sicker persons, politically negotiated and post hoc cost increases, shifting of costs to noncovered payers, substitution of complex services for conventional services, inability to differentiate serious disease (often afflicting the frail elderly) from milder impairment, the potential for profit-making facilities to skim off the more profitable clients, minimizing of losses through quicker discharges of patients, and unregulated expansion to additional medical services (Brown, 1983; *Health Advocate*, 1983–1984; Manheim, 1982; McClure, 1983; Tynan et al., 1981; Tyson & Merrill, 1983).

MEDICARE'S PROSPECTIVE PAYMENT SYSTEM

The cost containment revolution was climaxed between 1983 and 1985, according to some analysts, when the Medicare reimbursement system was changed from a cost-based retrospective approach to a fixed-price prospective method. Medicare's prospective payment system (PPS) was required in a few hospitals by October 1983. One year later 81% of Medicare hospitals were operating under PPS (Oriol, 1985), with the remainder joining over the next couple of years. The PPS formula is based on 468 categories of illness called diagnosis related groups (DRGs), into which each hospital patient's condition is classified. Each DRG is assigned a fixed payment level, which reflects the cost of treating an average patient for an average length of stay within a specific diagnostic category. Thus, regardless of the actual costs for treating a specific illness or disability, there is a predetermined payment rate. Some exceptions and variations do exist. There are a limited number of "outlier" patients whose illnesses require longer or more complex care than is covered within a single DRG. Also, hospital payments vary by their urban or rural location, wages in their area, and number of full-time interns and residents they employ.

Medicare's prospective payment system reached full implementation in 1988, when DRG payment rates were based on national averages rather than a combination of national and regional DRG payments and each hospital's history of costs. The full conversion may affect public hospitals and teaching/research facilities more adversely than for-profit hospitals if the higher percentage of charitable cases and the extra funds needed for educational and research purposes are not adequately taken into consideration (Tyson & Merrill, 1983). In addition, hospitals differ widely on their case mix, which depends on types of people served, types of services offered, intensity of services required, complexity of cases, and other factors. The DRG formula must remain responsive to a specific hospital's case mix or inequities will occur (Dunham & Morone, 1983).

There are problems that fall outside of formula adjustments, however, such as making diagnostic categories clear enough to allow patient data to fit consistently into appropriate groups, developing the staff capacity to collect and analyze data, mollifying physicians who must transfer much of their decisionmaking authority to hospital administrators and government officials, convincing patients they are being discharged for medical reasons and not for financial considerations, and shifting costs to patients who are not covered under the prospective payment system.

HEALTH MAINTENANCE ORGANIZATIONS

Health maintenance organizations (HMOs) are prepaid medical organizations with fixed budgets that rely on incentives or controls to contain costs. The principal mode of cost containment is tighter control over the allocation of expensive medical resources, especially hospitalization. Studies show, for instance, that hospitalization rates are dramatically lowered by HMOs (about 59%) even when demographic characteristics such as age and health status are controlled (U.S. General Accounting Office, 1981).

Other characteristics of HMOs that are associated with lower costs are the reduction of unnecessary surgery, medical tests, and other expensive health care services; use of nonphysician personnel for standard procedures such as routine examinations, medical histories, and immunizations; and less complex claim filing procedures.

Another aspect of cost containment through HMOs is a greater emphasis on health promotion, preventive health care, and early disease detection. Many HMOs provide coverage or referral for health care screenings, routine physical examinations, exercise classes, nutrition education, stress management programs, self-care instruction, smoking cessation and alcohol/chemical abuse programs, and weight control classes. A survey of HMOs in the Washington Metropolitan area revealed that while a majority of the plans provided or referred members to health programs and paid part or all of the cost, some plans did not follow up on their claims to provide prevention and promotion programs (*Checkbook,* 1986).

In general, enrollees in HMOs can take advantage of health programs and, in addition, may change health attitudes and adopt health-promoting behaviors. The cost-effectiveness of such activities in terms of disease prevention or lower use of medical services is not easily documented because most evaluations fail to use control groups, separate the program impact from other confounding influences, or examine long-term effects (Business and health, 1985).

Another way in which HMOs differ from traditional fee-for-service programs is the more versatile quality control programs. Many of these programs use computer printouts to allow physicians to compare number and type of prescriptions written, number and type of laboratory tests and X rays ordered, and number of days patients with the same diagnosis remain in the hospital. While HMOs subject physicians and other health care professionals to more oversight than fee-for-service programs, the extent to which these safeguards have real impact and are responsible for reducing expensive and unnecessary health care practices has not been adequately documented (*Checkbook,* 1986).

HMO cost savings, according to one study, do not appear to be achieved through the hiring of lower quality physicians, as alleged by opponents of the HMO system. A comparison of nine HMOs in the Washington Metropolitan area with fee-for-service plans reveals that the HMOs have more board certified physicians and the same percentage of graduates from more demanding U.S. medical schools as do the fee-for-service plans (*Checkbook,* 1986).

In general, HMOs provide more services at lower costs to enrollees. Nonetheless, there are potential drawbacks. HMO participants are limited in their choice of physicians, the location of services may be less convenient, access to world renowned specialization centers may be denied, enrollees may find that the process of switching physicians or leaving an HMO is more time-consuming than they like, physicians paid on a capitation basis (a uniform stipend per patient regardless of the number of visits) instead of a salary basis may discourage patient access to them, physicians may be offered incentives to limit the use of specialists, and physicians may underserve clients if they are vulnerable to financial risks when costs elevate above the collective premium level (Hornbrook, 1983).

A system akin to HMOs that does not place physicians at financial risk is the preferred provider organization (PPO). PPOs make agreements with fee-for-service providers who are willing to deliver services at discount rates in exchange for large numbers of patients and prompt payments (Ginsburg, 1983; McClure, 1983). Rather than placing physicians at financial risk, cost control is attained by dropping physicians if their costs are excessive (Pierce & Hekman, 1983). Physicians are more willing to conform to the lower rate schedules required by PPOs because of a surplus of doctors competing for patients (Tyson & Merrill, 1983). Patients are motivated to the use PPOs because they have greater freedom to choose providers than the standard HMO program. Also, since PPOs need not be organizations per se, but merely agreements with providers covering utilization controls, claims procedures, and payment arrangements, they are easier and less expensive to operate than HMOs (Fox et al., 1984).

The fine line between HMOs and PPOs is beginning to blur, however, as HMOs adopt some of the positive features of the PPOs. HMO enrollees in some plans, for instance, may use nonparticipating providers if enrollees assume greater responsibility for cost sharing. As HMOs, PPOs, and other prepaid plans become more complex, it becomes more difficult for consumers to evaluate the relative merits of the plans in terms of cost containment and quality of care.

HMO GROWTH

In 1971 the federal government began issuing grants and loan guarantees to support the establishment of health maintenance organizations on a widespread basis. After a decade of struggle, though, financial aid to HMOs was phased out (Brown, 1983), with the HMO movement having expanded from 2% of the population in 1971 to only 4% in 1981. Beginning in the 1980s, however, the growth of HMOs throughout the country accelerated and is beginning to approach the medical care transformation once envisioned by government officials. There were 11.6 million HMO enrollees in 1982 (Ginsburg, 1983), 19 million in 1985 (Abramowitz, 1986), and a projected growth to 30 million by 1990 (Fox et al., 1984).

Grants and loans to HMOs were unsuccessful in the 1970s because the era of cost containment was not quite in vogue. By the late 1970s to early 1980s, however, both government officials and private sector leaders acknowledged the urgent need for health care cost containment practices. While government officials were dismayed by accelerating costs of the Medicare and Medicaid programs, there were similar concerns in the private sector. Collectively, firms were paying $90 billion a year for health care premiums for their workers (Rich, 1985a). Chrysler Corporation, to cite a specific example, discovered that $530 was added on to the cost of every car sold in 1984 because of employee health care plans alone (Rich, 1985a).

One response to the need for cost containment in the government sector was the 1982 Tax Equity and Fiscal Responsibility Act, by which the Medicare program was granted the authority to negotiate contracts with federally accredited HMOs to provide service to Medicare enrollees on a group basis. It was hoped that these Medicare HMOs would save the government money in two ways. First, the HMOs' fixed, monthly, prepaid premium rate was set at 95% of the amount the government would be expected to pay through its regular Medicare program. Thus the government expected to save 5% of its costs. Second, the federal government hoped to save money on the processing of individual claims for service through the payment of one predetermined sum to the Medicare HMO. A third means of saving money could occur through use of prevention and promotion services by elderly enrollees.

The cost savings by Medicare HMOs has not yet been documented. The potential for growth, however, is indisputable. Nearly 1 million Medicare beneficiaries signed on with 1 of the 150 participating HMOs by September of 1987 (Polich & Iversen, 1987). This represents 3% of all Medicare beneficiaries throughout the United States, with over 50% of this growth taking place in 1986 and the first half of 1987. Older converts are attracted to HMO Medicare plans because beneficiaries do not have to pay deductibles and additional out-of-pocket expenses are small (typically limited to a $15 to $20 monthly membership fee) (Quinn, 1985). HMO services may be expanded to include eyeglasses, prescription drugs, and routine physical examinations, none of which are covered by the traditional Medicare plan. Other attractive features of the Medicare HMO plan to consumers are the reduced risk of unnecessary surgery and the avoidance of excessive claim filing (*Checkbook,* 1986). An early report from the Health Care Financing Administration notes that Medicare HMOs are attracting significant numbers of Medicare beneficiaries, and disenrollment rates are less than 5% (Ochsner, 1983).

In 1982 the federal government permitted states to set up their own requirements for HMO and PPO eligibility for Medicaid recipients. State Medicaid programs hoped to use HMOs and PPOs to exclude high-cost providers as well as constrain excessive users of service (Ronan, 1982). Some state officials believe that mandatory Medicaid prepayment programs encourage a more systematic approach to health care and discourage patient use of more expensive services, such as emergency room services. To make these programs mandatory, some state legislatures are repealing or altering their "freedom of choice" laws that require consumers to have free choice of providers, regardless of cost. California, for instance, has changed its state law to permit Medicaid recipients and private payers to pursue selective contracting arrangements through PPOs (National Governor's Association, 1984). In 1984, eight states considered bills to eliminate restrictions on the development and operation of PPOs (National Conference of State Legislators, 1984).

While older persons continue to join Medicare and Medicaid prepayment plans in steadily increasing numbers, there are several significant issues that still need to be addressed. For instance, older persons are more likely to have established a long-standing relationship with a physician and may be more reluctant to give up their primary practitioners for those who are associated with an HMO plan (Newcomer et al., 1983). Also there have been reported difficulties with leaving an HMO plan in an expeditious manner when a specialist outside of the plan is desired (Quinn, 1985).

From the perspective of the HMO, several have experienced substantial losses due to their inability to predict the frailty level of new members and the resulting increase in expenditure patterns (Ochsner, 1983). This problem, referred to as adverse selection, occurs when a disproportionate percentage of Medicare enrollees requires medical services. The negative impact of adverse selection may be even greater in the future when Medicare HMO enrollees no longer tend to be healthier than the general Medicare population. Current Medicare HMO enrollees have less need for medical care and have lower mortality rates (Quinn, 1985).

In the private sector the current success of HMOs may also be due to the avoidance of adverse selection. HMOs can locate in growing suburbs where a younger, healthier mix of enrollees is located. The HMO plan may offer services, such as well baby care, that attract a younger, lower risk group of persons (Luft, 1985). Thus, HMOs may focus on higher profits rather than a philosophy of providing more appropriate medical care at lower costs (Winsberg, 1985). The more established HMOs, however, may be stuck with older employees, who are more vulnerable to chronic illness (Levin, 1987).

The growth of HMOs and PPOs in the future will be dependent on adequate computer software programs and responsible management policies. Government and private sector prepaid programs will need to know what type of patient mix can include the older, more vulnerable participant, while still allowing for a profit. Also HMOs and PPOs need to document which physicians are practicing efficiently and which are not, thereby eliminating unnecessary services while retaining quality of care. Thus, a good data processing system is essential to the success of an HMO or PPO (Abramowitz, 1986).

REGULATORY RESTRUCTURING

While the caveat "let the buyer beware" may be appropriate in other competitive arenas, the contemporary American medical system is too complex for untrained consumers to negotiate. Thus, we have a system where the provider determines whether a product or service is needed, what type of health care will be delivered, and how much of it is necessary. Given the imbalance of power between the provider and the consumer, most analysts suggest that government regulation is needed to protect the consumer's interest. Regulatory systems, however, have been impeded by limited financial resources, political and legal constraints, limited data on decisionmaking, and unclear objectives (cost containment versus quality of care) (Eustis et al., 1984).

Two major regulatory systems evolved from the National Health Planning and Resources Development Act of 1974, which (1) required all states to establish certificate of need (CON) programs and (2) funded 204 health systems agencies (HSAs) to plan health services and contain costs.

State CON programs require health care facilities to justify capital expenditures over a certain amount of money, change in bed capacity, and additions to the existing range of services provided (Feder & Scanlon, 1980). While not all states are enthusiastic supporters of the certificate of need concept, most agree that the programs are necessary and should be retained. Several studies support this view, especially in reference to restricting the number of hospital beds and the growth of new technology (Feder et al., 1982; Cook et al., 1983).

Furthermore, CONs would counteract the unintended effects of changes in reimbursement rates. In New York State, for example, state reimbursement levels were liberalized and the supply of nursing home beds exceeded what state officials felt the state could afford (Tynan et al., 1981). A more restrictive CON policy, however, slowed the expansion to an acceptable level. This strategy controlled the growth of health care facilities and technological expansion throughout the country during the 1960s and the 1970s (Ginsburg, 1983; Tynan et al., 1981).

By the early 1980s, however, research data suggested that CON programs were not having much impact on cost containment. CONS were being circumvented in nursing homes, for instance, in a number of ways: by the reallocation of funds to unregulated items like nursing home staff and other service-intensified expenditures; by limiting the nursing home bed supply so that operators could afford to restrict Medicaid patients, overly demanding patients, and others who were backed up inappropriately and at considerable expense in hospitals; and by stifling competition so that there was considerable disregard of licensing standards by many existing nursing homes that were protected from competition (Feder & Scanlon, 1980; Pierce & Hekman, 1983; Sloan, 1983; U.S. General Accounting Office, 1982). Thus, by 1983 an increasing number of states allowed their CON regulations to lapse or placed moratoriums on certain types of CON applications (Pierce & Hekman, 1983). Also the Reagan administration increasingly removed CON programs from federal guidelines or sanctions.

Regarding health systems agencies, a nationwide network was set up to plan health services and to contain health care costs. Perhaps the major contribution of the HSAs to date has been the expansion of an experienced nationwide cadre of local health planners and the collection and analysis of vital data on health care use and quality (Goldbeck, 1984). As a change-inducing agent, however, the review and recommendation powers granted to HSAs were ineffectual, according to several reports. The U.S. Comptroller General (1981), for example, cites that most HSA plans were unmeasurable, unrealistic, and overabundant. Also, either the goals to be implemented through the plans were unstated, or there were insufficient resources to accomplish them (Pegels, 1980). Since 1981 federal funding for health planning has been severely reduced, and many states have abolished HSAs (Atchley, 1985).

The Social Security Amendments of 1972 established another regulatory structure, professional standards review organizations (PSROs). PSROs were local, state, and regional nonprofit organizations staffed by physicians for the purpose of determining the appropriateness of Medicare and Medicaid admissions to hospitals, the length of hospital stays, and the quality of professional standards being implemented.

The major concerns with PSROs were that the nationwide network of 195 organizations cost more than it was worth; that the organizations were unfocused, attempting to assess quality and contain costs at the same time; that staffing PSROs with physicians and hospital administrators placed the foxes in charge of the chicken coop; that a system more appropriate in a hospital setting was transferred inappropriately to the nursing home setting; and that government financial support never matched the operational requirements needed to achieve the objectives (Congressional Budget Office, 1979; Fox et al., 1984; Kane et al., 1979; Smits, 1981).

On the other hand, some analysts suggested that PSROs did deter the growth of health costs, though many of these accomplishments went unnoticed because of inadequate measurement tools (Smits, 1981; Tierney et al., 1982). Moreover, proponents of the PSRO process suggested that the model provided a clinical sophistication that could more accurately assess the process by which diseases are assigned to appropriate diagnostic groupings—a function that could be useful to Medicare's prospective payment system.

Because of the mixed reviews that discuss the impact of the PSRO, however, and the antiregulatory environment fostered by the Reagan administration, the 195 PSROs were replaced in 1984 by 52 statewide peer review organizations (PROs) (see Appendix A). Unlike the PSROs, which merely received government grants and were not performance-judged organizations, the PROs must compete for government contracts and, most likely, will need to attract the private sector to survive (Fox et al., 1984).

The PROs have a more clearly defined mandate than previous attempts at regulation. In comparison to PSROs, which disciplined only 70 physicians and hospitals between 1978 and 1984, the PROs have begun proceedings against 950 doctors, mostly for poor care, and 183 hospitals, primarily for costly and unnecessary treatment. The PRO also serves the older person by reviewing whether the hospital treatment was appropriate and whether quality care was provided. (See Fig. 1.1.) Sophisticated software is currently being developed to identify provider or facility inefficiency so that the PROs have the potential to reduce reimbursement rates accordingly (Fox et al., 1984).

In addition, the Health Care Financing Administration issued regulations in 1985 to allow PROs to collect data on measures of hospital quality and to make the data available to the public on a hospital-by-hospital basis. Potential customers can now access data relating to mortality rates, postoperative infection rates, surgical volume (which directly correlates with surgery success rates), and other indicators of quality care and cost (Business and health, 1985). The science of determining quality care in hospitals, however, is not yet definitive. Hospital-specific mortality data published in a six-volume issue of the *Federal Register* (Office of Human Development Services, 1987) generated criticism from hospitals, which view such data as poor indicators of quality care. Existing mortality data does not consider such variables as the hospital's patient mix or the caring attitude of staff and does consider mortality after hospital discharge even though it may be unrelated to the medical condition for which the patient was admitted.

COMPETITION STRATEGIES

At first glance, competition in the health care arena does not seem particularly appropriate. According to the Office of State Health Planning (1982),

> *There are some roles in society which the private sector does not have the obligation, the interest, the incentives, nor the ability to play. Those roles are and should be public responsibilities. To expect private initiative to fulfill them is unfair to the private sector, and betrays a lack of understanding of the purpose of government in a complex industrial and technological society.*

Patient Checklist

BEFORE CHECKING INTO THE HOSPITAL. . .

☐ **Ask your doctor if the prescribed treatment could be safely and effectively administered on an outpatient basis.**

☐ **Begin to calculate what your estimated out-of-pocket hospital costs will be.** As soon as you know you may be admitted to the hospital, discuss with your doctor your treatment options and anticipated length of stay. Based upon this, you should be able to estimate your costs, including the first-day deductible and coinsurance payments after 60 days. Remember to include costs for items and services not covered by Medicare such as telephone and television fees.

☐ **Enlist your physician's help.** Ask your physician to explain to you and your family how the *Prospective Payment System* can be expected to affect your care in the hospital.

☐ **Consider asking someone to assist you.** You may decide to have a friend or relative available to make inquiries on your behalf should it be necessary while you are in the hospital. This person should be familiar with the material in this booklet.

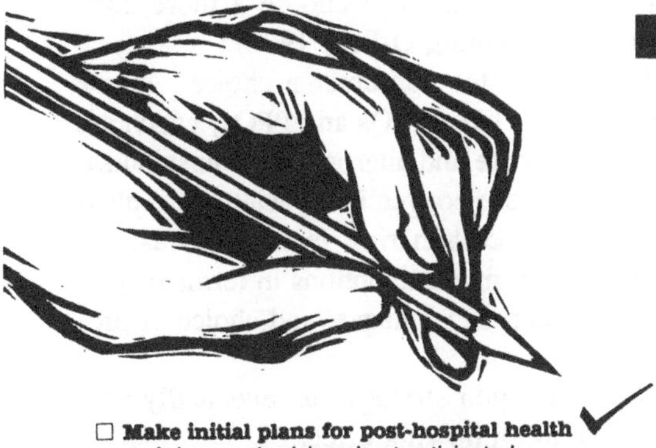

☐ **Make initial plans for post-hospital health care.** Ask your physician about anticipated care/treatment options that may be necessary after discharge from the hospital. For example, ask if you will be able to go directly home or if you will need nursing home care or home health care services following hospitalization. Prearrange for the services you may need after being discharged. Check on the cost of services and whether Medicare will pay for the services you'll need when you leave the hospital.

PF3602(885)

☐ **Look over your private insurance policy.** See what it does or doesn't cover. Most people are surprised to find that both Medicare and their supplemental insurance policies provide very limited coverage for nursing home or home health care.

UPON ENTERING THE HOSPITAL. . .

☐ **Be sure to take this booklet** with you for information on the PRO review process.

☐ **Read everything you sign at admission,** especially financial and "informed consent" documents. The hospital staff should be able to answer any questions you have about these forms. Never sign anything you do not understand.

☐ **Find out who on the hospital staff handles discharge planning.** Identify who will be responsible for planning any other services you need when you are discharged from the hospital. Write down this person's telephone number for easy access during your hospital stay.

☐ **Keep the address and telephone number for the PRO in your area handy.** The address and telephone number for each PRO is provided with the list at the back of this booklet.

WHILE YOU ARE IN THE HOSPITAL. . .

☐ **For questions about medical treatment, contact your physician.** Your physician is the one who establishes the plan for your medical treatment, who decides when you should be discharged from the hospital, and who can make important recommendations about your care after you leave the hospital. Share any concerns as soon as possible.

☐ **For questions about nursing or other hospital services, contact the Registered Nurse (R.N.) responsible for your care.** Other hospital personnel who may be able to answer questions about hospital policy or nursing services include the hospital's nursing director, social services director or patient ombudsman.

☐ **If it is recommended by the hospital that you no longer need inpatient care,** you have the right to:

- receive written notice that you will be liable for services beginning on the third calendar day after your receipt of the notice;
- continue to receive care covered by Medicare for the two-day period before your liability begins;
- request an immediate review by the PRO.

☐ **Remember to keep copies of all documents and bills for your records.**

FIGURE 1.1 Patient checklist. Copyright 1988 by the American Association of Retired Persons. Reprinted with permission.

Most procompetition strategists, however, do not advocate a laissez-faire doctrine. Even the staunchest supporter of competition recognizes the necessary role of government in the licensure of providers, safety codes, antitrust suits, issues of equity, and so forth. Furthermore, a competition strategy requires some regulation for it to work in the contemporary health care marketplace. Some of the additional safeguards needed are (1) the availability of large numbers of providers to act without collusion; (2) a price mechanism that is responsive to consumers, even though determined by competing providers; (3) free market entry and exit by providers; (4) adequate education so that consumers can bear the consequences of their decisions; (5) employer and government assistance that is equally applied to all providers; (6) enforcement of standards regarding premiums, benefit packages, and catastrophic protection; and (7) a ceiling on tax exemptions to avoid favoring costlier health plans (Brown, 1983; McClure, 1983; Office of State Health Planning, 1982; and U.S. General Accounting Office, 1982).

In the early 1980s 82% of all consumers who obtained health insurance as an employment benefit had only one plan offered to them (U.S. General Accounting Office, 1982). Lack of competition led to the selection of more comprehensive coverage than many employees would have opted for if given a monetary incentive (or a health promotion incentive) to choose a more cost-effective health care plan (U.S. General Accounting Office, 1982).

The competition strategy, therefore, offers the consumer a choice. At one end of the spectrum are the cost-effective plans like HMOs and PPOs, which are prepaid, capitated plans that stress preventive care and alternatives to hospitalization. At the other end of the continuum are more conventional health care plans that offer more elaborate coverage and high cost-sharing features. Thus, the competition approach provides consumers with multiple options in terms of premiums and other cost-sharing mechanisms, benefit packages, and choice of providers.

According to Enthoven (1980), a competition strategy can eventually produce economic pressures that would have the following effect:

> *People would gradually change to more economical health plans. Less economical health plans would have to find more effective cost controls. Newly trained physicians in specialties in excess supply in a given area would find no health plans interested in contracting with them, and they would have to look for work in areas where their services were needed. Primary-care physicians would assume more responsibility for the total costs of care for their patients, and specialists whose costs were judged by such primary-care physicians to be excessive would find themselves obliged to negotiate lower fees in order to retain their referrals. Individual practice associations would tighten utilization controls and more carefully balance the specialty mix of their participating physicians to the needs of their enrolled populations. Prepaid group practices would continue to grow. (p. 133)*

For competitive pressures to link with cost-effective health care decisions there is a need for fixed employer and government contributions across provider plans. If consumers opt for more expensive plans, they must subsidize the costs out of pocket. Conversely, if consumers choose a less expensive plan, a tax-free refund within the deductible limits allowed would be returned to them (McClure, 1983).

Several problems are likely to arise with the competition strategy. For example, there is the potential for low-risk persons, such as healthy younger and middle-aged adults, to opt for cost-effective coverage and for high-risk persons, such as aging persons with multiple chronic conditions, to opt for more comprehensive coverage. Eventually the gap between the two groups could widen to the point where comprehensive coverage becomes too expensive to afford for all but the rich (Hereford, 1982).

Another problem is that consumers must gamble on selecting the right mix of services and costs. This choice must be made in the absence of objective information about potential health problems in the coming year and with limited ability to understand complicated insurance contracts and to make a sound decision on varying levels of coverage and expense. An additional problem is that the competition approach requires higher administrative costs associated with monitoring the competing plans and providing employee information on them (U.S. General Accounting Office, 1982).

While the Reagan administration promoted a procompetition stance, the model has been slow to develop for two reasons. First, it appears that procompetition approaches do not, ironically, reduce the federal regulatory burden on the health care industry. In actuality, regulatory legislation encouraging competition tends to substitute federal for state involvement in the regulatory process, in opposition to what the procompetition Reagan administration intended (Hereford, 1982). Second, providers are reluctant to give up the regulatory system when it has provided so much security and generosity in preference to the uncertainty of the marketplace (Ginsburg, 1983).

CONCLUSION

In contrast to the multiplicity of programs, facts, and ideas touched on in this chapter, the conclusion can be condensed to two sentences.

The high cost, institutional-oriented, medically intensive health care system of the past few decades is only beginning to come to terms with the need for health care cost containment. Thus, the parallel and belated recognition of the need for widespread, community-based, chronic care services (which will be summarized in the next chapter) must be viewed from the onset in the sobering context of a cost containment framework.

2

ADDITIONAL CHALLENGE OF LONG-TERM CARE

AGING AMERICANS AND THE PLIGHT OF OLDER WOMEN

While demographers and gerontologists have focused considerable attention on the chronological age marker of 65, the original choice of this number to signify entry into old age in America was made by political analysts. A small group of youthful New Dealers was charged with the responsibility of drafting a landmark piece of legislation that would result in the Social Security Act of 1935. During the early 1930s these youthful New Dealers were very much aware that Congress would be more influenced by political considerations than by scientific research in the subsequent debate over the proposed legislation. Thus the decision to select age 65 as the age of eligibility for Social Security benefits was not based on research findings about the dwindling physical or mental capacity of aging persons to fulfill job responsibilities. Instead the decision was based on the need to remove a sufficiently large number of potential workers from the ranks of the unemployed—which at that time comprised about 25% of those of working age. In one bold initiative, therefore, older persons were removed from competition for scarce jobs, and 65 became the age of eligibility for Social Security benefits, the de facto marker for retirement, and the quantifiable onset of old age.

From a demographical perspective, age 65 has proved to be quite useful as a way of characterizing the growth of the so-called elderly population in America. Focusing on this segment of the population since the turn of the century, for

TABLE 2.1 Actual and Projected Growth of the Older Population, 1900–2050 (Numbers in Thousands)

Year	Total population all ages	65 years and over	
		Number	Percent
1900	76,303	3,084	4.0
1910	91,972	3,950	4.3
1920	105,711	4,933	4.7
1930	122,775	6,634	5.4
1940	131,669	9,019	6.8
1950	150,697	12,270	8.1
1960	179,323	16,560	9.2
1970	203,302	19,980	9.8
1980	226,505	25,544	11.3
1990	249,731	31,799	12.7
2000	267,990	35,036	13.1
2010	283,141	39,269	13.9
2020	296,339	51,386	17.3
2030	304,339	64,345	21.1
2040	307,952	66,643	21.6
2050	308,856	67,061	21.7

From the U.S. Bureau of the Census (1982). Decennial censuses of population, 1900–1980 and projections of the population of the United States: 1982 to 2050 (Advance Report). *Current Population Reports* (Series P-25), 922. Projections are middle series.

example, has revealed the inexorable "graying of America," from 4% in 1900 to 12.7% in 1990, to a projected 22% by the year 2050 (see Table 2.1).

From the perspective of analysts and policymakers involved with long-term care in the 1980s and beyond, however, the age 65 marker has not proved to be the most useful indicator of old age. Persons between the ages of 65 and 75, for instance, do not generate much demand for long-term care services. In contrast, it is the very old, those over age 85, who not only constitute the fastest growing segment of the population (See Fig. 2.1), but are the most dependent on long-term care services. A few statistics help demonstrate this point.

Persons age 85 and over in the community are about six times more dependent on others for assistance with basic or instrumental activities of daily living (Oriol, 1985). Basic activities are defined as eating, dressing, grooming, walking, bathing, getting in and out of bed, and continence. Instrumental activities include travel, shopping, preparing meals, housework, taking medicine, and managing money. Forty percent of those age 85 and over, for instance, need help with walking, while only 5% of those between ages 65 and 74 need such help (Califano, 1986). Twenty-two percent of those age 85 and over are in nursing homes, compared to only 1.5% of those age 65 to 74 (Califano, 1986).

The very old are not only more dependent but also are increasing in number more rapidly than other age groups. Between 1960 and 2000 the absolute number of persons age 65 and over will nearly double, but the number of persons age 85 and over will triple. Those who need the most services—the very old, age 85 and over—will increase from 6% of the elderly population to 10.4% during this period (Atchley, 1985). America is not just aging; the aged are aging too.

The aging of the aged is only half the picture needed to comprehend the long-term care needs of the future. Understanding gender differences with age is equally important. The Older Women's League, an advocacy, educational and support group focusing on women's issues nationwide, refers to long-term care as primarily a women's issue. Looking at the data, we find there is support for their claim. The most striking inequity is that four out of five informal *caregivers* in the community are women, and three out of four *care recipients* in long-term care institutions are women (Haber, 1986b). In other words, it is the woman's role to do the difficult tasks associated with informal caregiving in the community; but due to factors such as female longevity and societal age norms for marriage, women disproportionately are forced to accept assistance from the less desirable institutional setting. To add insult to the gender's injury, the underpaid aides who provide over 90% of all direct services in the nursing home are women as well.

Since the plight of aging women is exacerbated by unequal life expectancies and the burdensome custom of marrying older men, the obvious choice of caretaker when disability strikes—the spouse—is denied to most women. At age

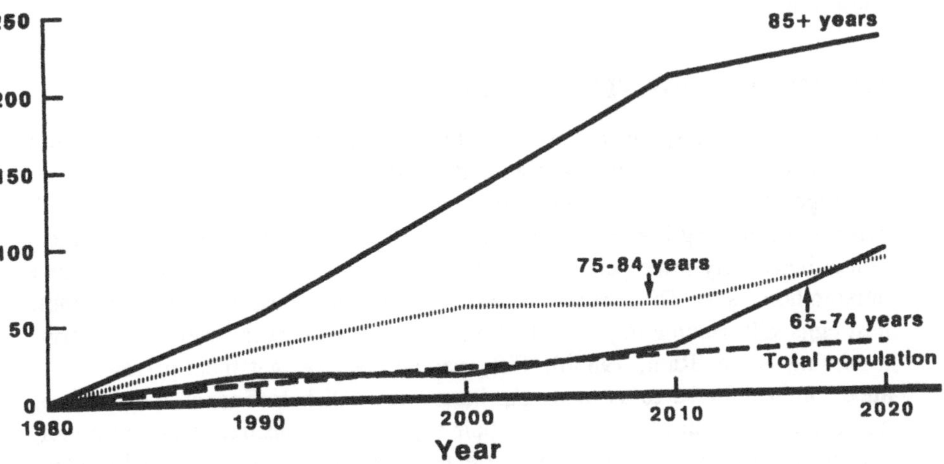

FIGURE 2.1 Projected change in elderly population: United States, 1980–2020 (percent change). From Nostrand, J. F. (1984). *The elderly LTC population, demographics and projections.* Primer session at the National Conference on the Complex Cube of LTC. Reprinted with permission from American Health Planning.

75 only 20% of women are married, while almost 70% of men are still living with their spouses (Oriol, 1985). When women turn to their next choice of caretaker, adult daughters and sisters, they find these caregivers are also aging and many have aging spouses to support. The caregiving situation is further threatened by several trends: The pool of adult children who are potential caregivers is shrinking, women are increasingly entering the work force, families are increasingly disrupted by divorce and separation, residential mobility within extended families is on the rise, and female caregivers are more often part of the sandwich generation—with caregiving responsibilities to both older and younger generations.

Another complication is that while caregiving is a very important role option for women in our society, informal caregivers still are not eligible for Social Security benefits. They are unlikely to qualify for public or private pension benefits and do not receive disability protection (Older Women's League, 1985). Not surprisingly, therefore, over 80% of the elderly poor are women (Older Women's League, 1985). Thus, a woman's capacity to afford homemaking services, home health aides, personal care, respite care, or any of a number of support services for herself during old age is diminished or nonexistent. For those in the triple jeopardy of being an older black woman, resources become even more meager with age. Older black women are three times more likely than older white women to live in poverty and five times more likely than older white men (Older Women's League, 1985).

In short, to tackle the problems of long-term care in America today, the aging of aged women must be acknowledged and the interventions designed appropriately.

MYTHS OF LONG-TERM CARE

A national survey sponsored by the American Association of Retired Persons (Hagan, 1984) revealed widespread and erroneous beliefs about long-term care coverage. Seventy-nine percent, for example, believe that Medicare will finance their nursing home stay, despite the reality that it provides scant protection at best. Fifty-three percent believe that earnings and savings will finance a nursing home stay. Those surveyed do not realize that most persons with sizable nest eggs still become impoverished within months, or even weeks, of entering a nursing home (Rich, 1985b). Fifty percent believe that their private insurance, often referred to as medi-gap insurance, will help finance their nursing home stay. They are unaware that their supplemental insurance policy merely fills in the gaps of the acute care-oriented Medicare coverage. Finally, while Medicaid does cover long-term care, it is an unacceptable alternative for most persons because it first requires that they become destitute.

As long as these widespread misconceptions persist, the development of long-term care alternatives will be hampered. It is not only important to analyze the deficiencies of existing long-term care programs and resources, therefore, but to disseminate this information in an effective manner. This latter task is difficult. The younger the targeted audience, the more remote the problem is. The older the audience, the fewer the options that can be developed. Also, many elected officials tend to advocate short-sighted solutions to long-term care problems to produce results within 2-, 4-, or 6-year periods, depending on their tenure in office.

MEDICARE MYTH

It is important to examine what Medicare is (hospital care and physician care for acute illness) and what it is not (long-term care).

Medicare is a federal program that was enacted in 1965 to provide health insurance for the elderly and the disabled. Medicare is financed through Social Security payroll deductions, individual contributions, and federal subsidy. Part A is hospital insurance, and it pays primarily for inpatient hospital care and limited skilled nursing care. Part B is supplementary medical insurance, and it pays for a portion of the physician's fee, tests, therapies, and medical equipment. About one-quarter of Part B is paid for through premiums, deductibles, and copayments; the remainder is picked up by the American taxpayer.

Medicare does not cover chronic care needs such as eyeglasses, dental services, foot care, outpatient drugs, hearing aids, physical examinations, immunizations (with one exception), outpatient psychiatric care (beyond $250), or any type of illness prevention or health promotion services. Only 4% of the Medicare budget spent on care for the elderly went for long-term care in skilled nursing facilities or in home care services. While the home care program is the fastest growing component of Medicare, it is still limited to acute care needs and constitutes only 3% of expenditures (Oriol, 1985).

Over the years Medicare has been an unqualified success in providing older Americans access to acute health care in the hospital and promoting greater use of physician services. Seven years before Medicare, for instance, 32% of the age 65 and over segment of the population did not see a physician. Five years after its implementation this proportion was reduced to 24% (Aday et al., 1980). Medicare pays for the benefits of 30 million Americans, 90% of whom are elderly (Oriol, 1985).

Unfortunately, Medicare has been very successful with consuming an increasing amount of the federal budget as well. From 1967 to 1984 Medicare rose from less than 3% of the federal budget to more than 7% (Califano, 1986). Among domestic programs it is second only to Social Security in the magnitude of its expenditures. Medicare covers 75% of the hospital bills of beneficiaries and provides 30% of all hospital revenues; similarly, it covers over half of the physician bills of beneficiaries and provides over 20% of physician revenues (Califano, 1986).

One way to meet the expense of such a mammoth program is to increase the cost-sharing burden of beneficiaries. This already has been done to a substantial degree. In 1986 (some 1988 revisions will be examined later) the deductible on a hospital admission increased from $400 to $492. At the 60th inpatient day there was a $123 daily copayment; at the 90th day, $246 daily; at the 250th day, total costs were borne by the patient. Upon entering a skilled nursing home, the Medicare beneficiary paid $61.50 a day after the 20th day of residency. Part B required monthly premiums ($17.90), copayments (at least 20% of physician charges), and an annual deductible ($75). Also the majority of the elderly pay extra charges beyond the reasonable or customary charges that Medicare allows. As a result, the elderly today spend a higher percentage of their annual income on medical care than before Medicare was enacted (National Council on the Aging, 1982).

As Medicare continues to consume ever larger percentages of the federal budget and the older person's income because of acute care needs alone, the Medicare legislative agenda has been reluctant to move into the long-term care arena.

MEDICAID MYTH

Unlike Medicare, Medicaid is designed to fund the health care of the poor, including the elderly poor. Also unlike Medicare, the Medicaid program is not an insurance program partially funded through payroll contributions. It is a federal and state program based on general revenues to fund the health care needs of poor Americans with low income levels and few assets. The federal contribution, which ranges from 50% to 78% depending on the per capita income of the state, does include some general guidelines for state officials. State governments can vary among themselves, however, in program eligibility and types of services offered.

The emphasis on health care for the poor and the unique federal-state partnership are not the only distinctive features of the Medicaid program. It is also the primary public subsidy for long-term care in America. Thus, while Medicaid is directed to all the poor, not just the elderly, its long-term care objective assures that a disproportionate percentage of expenditures are targeted to the frail elderly. Given the institutional bias of this program (similar to the Medicare bias, which targets hospital care), a sizable amount of federal and state Medicaid monies goes toward nursing home care for residents who are overwhelming elderly (about 90%).

As one might expect for a program designed exclusively for low-income persons, Medicaid has not been lavish with its benefits nor, until recently, innovative in shaping the long-term care direction of the country. In fact, the Medicaid program has always been in danger of establishing a two-tiered health care system. In the long-term care arena this means better nursing home care and a variety of community-based options are only available to those who can afford to privately finance them. For the Medicaid recipient, though, there is impoverishment, substandard nursing home care, and few options for long-term care in the community. For the near-poor who do not qualify for Medicaid benefits there are no long-term care options in the public sector.

From the perspective of Medicaid recipients and those who were bumped from Medicaid eligibility, life became more difficult in the early 1980s. The New Federalism policies of the Reagan administration were an attempt to shift responsibility for domestic programs from the federal to the state government. The state governments, however, were already spending more on their state Medicaid programs than they deemed prudent in light of the total state revenues being received (National Conference of State Legislatures, 1984). The situation worsened with the New Federalism policy. From 1981 to 1983 the states' shares of Medicaid expenditures increased 22% while tax revenues rose only 14% (Newcomer et al., 1983). In response, 36 states adopted proposals in 1981 and 1982 alone to restrict Medicaid eligibility or to limit or eliminate services. By the mid-1980s about 25% of those classified as poor by the federal government were ineligible for Medicaid benefits, even though Medicaid allegedly remained a program for the poor. For those who continued to be covered, there were fewer service benefits and more copayments.

A summary of state Medicaid cost-cutting strategies includes the following: enrolling recipients into health maintenance organizations, signing contracts with preferred providers, reimbursing Medicaid hospital costs through prospective payment systems and competitive contracting, limiting physician visits and hospital stays, adopting a prospective payment system to nursing homes, and initiating copayments on prescription drugs. By 1988 all of these cost containment strategies were accelerating among state governments.

At the same time these cost containment measures were beginning to be enacted, the federal government encouraged community-based alternatives through the Omnibus Budget Reconciliation Act of 1981. This initiative, however, has been tentative and limited. Federal government officials have been concerned that community-based care options will add to the costs of institutional care rather than provide an alternative means of care. In addition to the potential for opening up a Pandora's box of consumer demand, it is difficult to determine how quality care in the community will be monitored and how costly it will be to administer. Thus, the major focus of the Medicaid program continues to be on controlling escalating costs rather than the radical restructuring of a health care system that needs to become more responsive to an aging society.

Over the past decade, the Medicare and Medicaid programs were major contributors to rising health care costs. By the early 1980s three fourths of the federal health care dollar was targeted to the Medicare and Medicaid programs. Between 1977 and 1984 hospital costs (three fourths of which were reimbursed by Medicare) and nursing home care costs (almost half of which were reimbursed through Medicaid) each rose about 15% *per year* (Waldo & Lazenby, 1984). Between 1981 and 1982 alone, health care goods and services increased from 9.8% of the Gross National Product to 10.5% (National Governor's Association, 1984).

GOOD FAMILY MYTH

Over half the persons in the survey sponsored by the American Association of Retired Persons believed that their earnings and saving could finance a nursing home stay or that their private insurance would help finance such a stay. Others believed that family members could provide the labor needed to maintain an elder at home, if necessary. Many of these personal beliefs, unfortunately, were premised not on financial capacity, but on the desire to conform to the myth that good families do not allow elders to be institutionalized. Typically, the family member proclaims, "My parent [sibling, grandparent, etc.] will never be forced to live in a publicly supported nursing home."

Earnings and savings, however, are spent within a matter of months or even weeks after the older person enters a nursing home through payment of private funds. Even those with sizable nest eggs tend to underestimate the cumulative and relentless costs involved with nursing home care. In about 13 weeks time, half the elderly entering a nursing home will exhaust their private savings (Rich, 1985b). By the end of 2 years, up to 91% will become destitute because of the high cost of nursing home care. The same length of time—about 2 years—impoverishes over half the families providing care at home to an Alzheimer's disease victim (Rich, 1985b).

Unbeknownst to many enrollees, private insurance or medi-gap insurance merely covers the acute care deductibles and copayments of the Medicare program. The highly effective advertising by popular television personalities who pitch the wares of medi-gap insurance inevitably omits the insurance program's inappropriate emphasis on acute care and institutionalization. Until sound actuarial estimates of long-term care costs can be calculated, however, private insurance companies will continue to remain hesitant about entering the nursing home or community-based long-term care insurance markets except on an experimental and limited basis. Given the size of the American Association of Retired Persons (AARP) organization (27 million in 1987) one of the most important long-term care insurance experiments is AARP's policy, which it began offering to members in 1987. By February 1988, 32,000 members had enrolled in its long-term care plan.

While these insurance experiments continue, families continue to meet long-term care crises with limited resources and without support or direction from a national long-term care policy. The absence of a national long-term care policy appears to work at some level since among people of equal impairment two to three manage to be cared for by families in the community for every one in a long-term institution. New policies, in fact, could reduce existing familial support or result in escalating government expenditures.

On the other hand, governmental incentive policies could be beneficial to families and need to be tested around the country. One set of incentives focuses on tax deductions, tax credits, direct payment to family members providing in-home care, and related economic policies (Arling & McAuley, 1983). The empirical question raised by these programs and yet to be definitively answered is whether they strengthen family support or weaken it. To what extent will economic assistance prolong or reinforce support? Under what circumstances will it replace the love and respect that drive most informal networks today?

Another set of incentives focuses on caregiver training and support programs for family members and community volunteers (Clark & Rakowsi, 1983; Montgomery & Prothero, 1985). While testimonials and nonrigorous evaluations demonstrate that these programs are useful for many participants, the evidence is not clear on how effective they are in terms of postponing or preventing institutionalization of the care recipient, maintaining the health and the supportive role of the caregiver, or producing other benefits that justify the costs of the program. Implementing these programs creates a set of questions that need answers. For example, will those in need of programs pay sufficient fees to subsidize the costs? If not, will government subsidized programs pay for themselves over the long term through reduced expenditures to institutional care? Is it even possible to evaluate the cost-effectiveness of training and support programs given the complexity of factors that can impinge on program outcomes? Regardless of cost-effectiveness, are the programs valued enough by society (i.e., taxpayers) to be subsidized?

From the perspective of a coercive policy, can government force families to care for elders either at home or in an institution? In 1983 Idaho (in addition to joining the list of states that provide incentive policies, such as tax deductions and credits for maintaining an elderly family member in the home) attempted to reduce its long-term care Medicaid budget by requiring financially capable children to contribute to their parents' nursing home expenses (Quinn, 1985). While the law was overturned, additional efforts in this regard will be tried. The danger of such a negative policy is that it might increase the resentment of children and weaken family ties. Also, this type of legislation might increase the dread (and the high suicide rate) of older persons who wish to avoid being a burden on their children. A more practical consideration is how such a program would be administered. Further, how would financial equity be determined when families differ on the basis of size, geographical proximity, competing obligations among members, intactness (divorced, remarried), income, and so forth?

Given the complexity of many existing programs, perhaps the absence of policy has been an adequate short-term solution. In the long run, however, the government will need to provide responsive leadership to the growing demand for community long-term care resources and the increasing limits on the capacity of family members to provide it by themselves.

NEED FOR CHRONIC CARE AT HOME OR IN THE COMMUNITY

Long-term care refers to the ongoing assistance needed by persons with a chronic illness or condition. In contemporary America, about 80% of this assistance is provided by the informal caregiving network—family, friends, neighbors, and volunteers from congregations and other community organizations. At the care level required of individuals who are eligible for long-term care institutional support, at least two of three persons currently receive informal caregiving at home or in the community. Thus, the strength of the caregiving network at home is more important for predicting whether someone will be institutionalized than the frailty level of the care recipient (Horowitz & Dobrof, 1982). The more durable and resourceful the informal network, the more likely that institutional placement can be postponed or avoided.

The future of community-based long-term care, however, is marked by obstacles. The three major challenges facing informal caregivers are (1) shrinking caregiving networks, (2) increasing numbers of debilitated elderly, and (3) a huge federal deficit and state budget problems that limit publicly financed resources and services. While these challenges are substantial, so is the motivational level of both family members and policymakers. Both prefer informal caregiving at home for economic and humanistic reasons. From an economic perspective, noninstitutional care is more cost-effective with all but the most severely impaired. From a humanistic perspective, the home provides greater self-determination, more privacy, and a more personalized decor. Nursing homes, in contrast, are not homes; they are institutions. Even the best ones are organized more for the efficiency of staff than for the individualized needs of residents.

Motivation alone is not sufficient to meet the challenges of the future. Innovative ideas for training caregivers, supporting them in the community, offering them respite, and encouraging their participation in health promotion programs must be developed, tested, and refined. At the same time, comprehensive long-term care policies and programs must be developed to be responsive to the tremendous variety of needs generated by unique caregiving situations. These new or revised programs must be more responsive than the current versions of Medicare, Medicaid, and other federal and state health and social service programs. Family members and grass roots community organizers cannot be expected to shoulder the burden alone. Federal and state governments must provide both direction and coordination of effort.

3

COMMUNITY-BASED LONG-TERM CARE

This chapter describes some of the alternatives being tested in community-based long-term care. The major issues weaving through these alternatives are accessibility or affordability and quality. In the era of health care cost containment it is often not clear whether a new approach to long-term care is motivated by controlling costs, shifting the burden of costs, or altering the quality of a given service. Complicating the matter is the confusing array of services and financial entitlements that serves the public instead of a coordinated comprehensive long-term care system. Given fragmented programs and confusing, even conflicting, objectives, it has been difficult to evaluate the effectiveness of individual programs.

CASE-MANAGED COMMUNITY CARE

Several community long-term care projects for the impaired elderly around the country have been subsidized through special waivers of Medicare or Medicaid regulations. These projects have waived ordinary rules of eligibility and benefits to offer alternative services at home or in the community. In addition to Medicare and Medicaid waivers, projects were often financed through Title XX, Older Americans Act, and state funds and included an evaluation component (Fig. 3.1).

Through the 1970s and 1980s these demonstration projects have focused on the same testable thesis: that the substitution of community care for nursing home care may be more appropriate and more cost-effective for elders at risk.

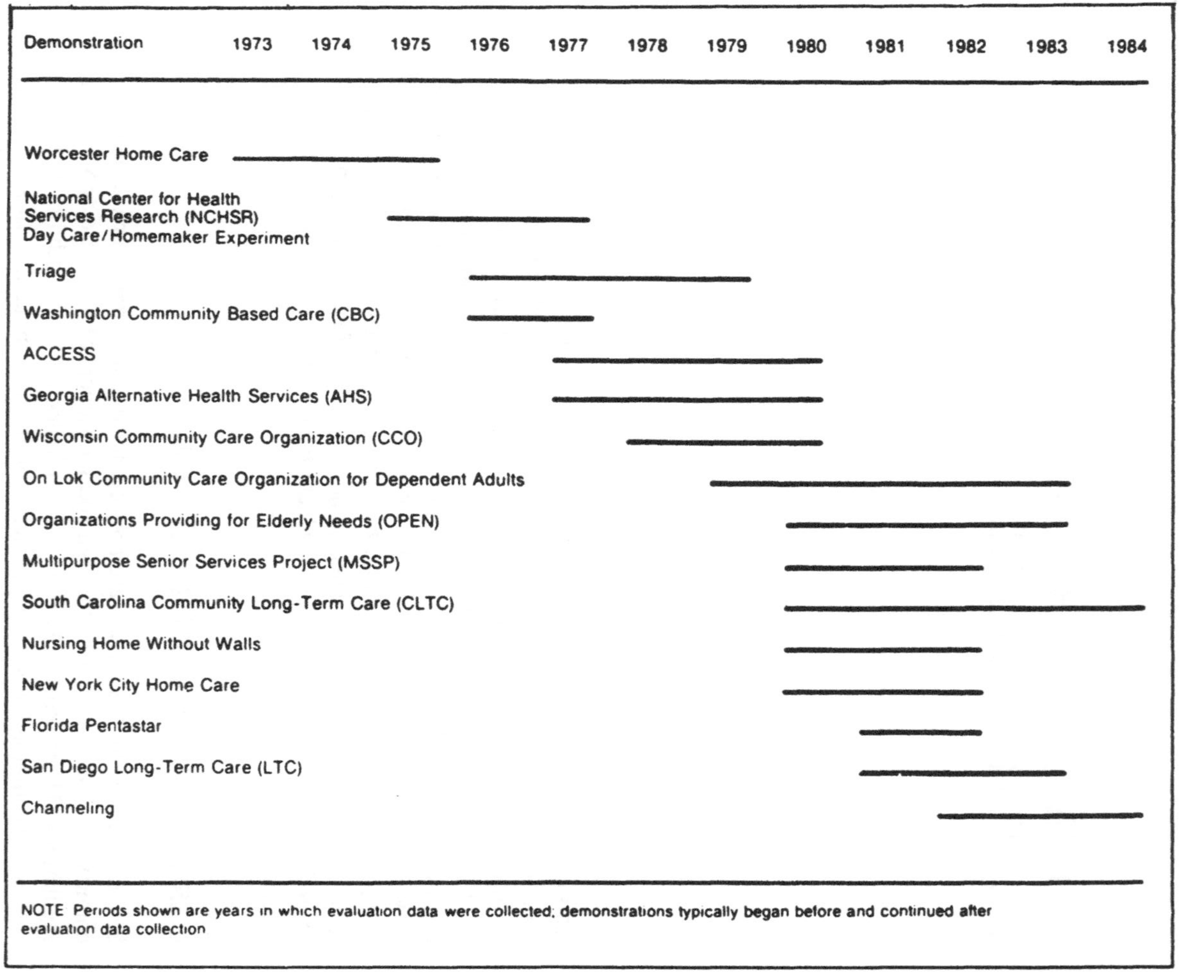

FIGURE 3.1 Timing of evaluation data collection by time period. From *Health Care Financing Review*. (1987), *8*(4), p.89. Reprinted with permission.

In addition, these projects share the same methodological components: (1) the examination of a case management element, which consists of needs assessments, design of care plans, coordination of services, and monitoring of client needs; and (2) the examination of an expanded array of community services, such as homemaker services, respite or adult day care, personal care (regardless of a need for skilled nursing care), transportation, home-delivered meals, and other nonmedical in-home services.

Typically these Medicare and Medicaid waiver projects have limited their expenditures on community service to 60% to 85% of nursing home reimbursement rates. They have also limited their client eligibility to only those persons who are at risk for nursing home placement. In addition, many of these programs have developed eligibility criteria for frail elderly that are based on the measurement of physical or mental disability or on demonstrated service needs. The most common measures of frailty were the activities of daily living (eating, bathing, dressing, etc.) and instrumental activities of daily living (transportation, cooking, etc.) indices. Finally, these programs tend to employ a methodology that compares those who were eligible for case management or expanded services and those in similar circumstances who were not eligible and were assigned to comparison groups.

As summarized by D. Kemper and associates (1987), Capitman (1986), and Capitman and associates (1986), there was no evidence that these community-based alternatives reduced nursing home use or overall costs in a statistically significant manner in comparison to control groups. Moreover, despite the attempt to measure frailty, subjects were generally *not* at risk of nursing home placement. Often this finding was demonstrated by the control group members who did not have the opportunity for expanded home care services and who still managed to stay in the community and avoid nursing homes.

Other findings from the demonstration projects, as summarized by D. Kemper and associates (1987), revealed that case managed services in the community did not change hospital utilization; did increase state and federal costs; did slightly reduce family responsibility for instrumental tasks (transportation, cooking, etc.) but did not necessarily improve the durability of informal caregivers; and did improve client life satisfaction, health functioning, and health status.

In summary, state and federal costs are likely to increase when there is public financing of community care alternatives. This is due primarily to the difficulty of identifying persons who would actually go into a nursing home in the absence of expanded community services. While many demonstration project clients were certifiably frail and eligible for nursing home care, they managed to avoid such an option regardless of their need. On the other hand, while rising costs are associated with community care programs, there are documentable benefits as well. The quality of life of older clients and caregivers is favorably impacted. Thus, the ultimate questions become: Under what circumstances, if any, does society value publicly financed community long-term care? How should it be financed? What services are to be provided? Who should benefit?

CHANNELING, SHMOs, AND THE CATASTROPHIC ACT

The most comprehensive and rigorous test of case managed community care programs was the "channeling project" or, more formally, the National Long Term Care Demonstration. The project was jointly funded by three units of the Department of Health and Human Services: Office of the Assistant Secretary for Planning and Evaluation, Administration on Aging, and Health Care Financing Administration. The channeling demonstration program was designed to identify, through screening, older clients who were at high risk of entering a nursing home. Clients were screened primarily on functional capacity and unmet service needs. Two models were tested. The basic case management model helped clients gain access to services and coordinated such services if provided by multiple sources (tested in Baltimore, Maryland; Eastern Kentucky; Houston, Texas; Middlesex County, New Jersey; and Southern Maine). The financial control model expanded community services that could be allocated to clients on the basis of need (tested in Cleveland, Ohio; Greater Lynn, Massachusetts; Miami, Florida; Philadelphia, Pennsylvania; Rensselaer County, New York). While services could be expanded, there were limits on expenditures. Individual public expenditures, for instance, could not exceed 85% of the average nursing home rate in the area; case managers were required to limit average expenditures for clients to 60% of the nursing home rate.

Almost 12,000 applicants were screened for the channeling demonstration program, with more than half of them randomly assigned to a treatment or a control group. The treatment group was assigned to either the basic case management or financial control model, and the control group continued to receive existing services, if available, in their community.

The results (Mathematica Policy Research, 1986) of channeling were consistent with the previously summarized studies:

1. Formal community service use increased, especially with the services most difficult to obtain—personal care and homemaker services.
2. Community services did not take the place of more costly nursing home placement.
3. Community services did not reduce informal caregiving, either in number of caregivers or amount of care given (except in limited ways under the financial control model, i.e., with friends and neighbors, not primary caregivers).
4. Community services did not affect hospitalization rates, utilization patterns with physicians, and use of other medical services.

In short, the costs associated with expanding case management and community services were not offset by reductions in nursing home costs or with hospital/physician/medical service use. Also, while health costs to clients and their families were reduced by 7%, government costs increased 14% under the basic case management model and 28% under the financial control model.

Channeling did have a positive impact on quality of life. It reduced unmet service needs and increased life satisfaction of clients and their informal caregivers. Channeling, however, did not go so far as to reduce mortality rates or improve client functioning.

Finally, reductions in nursing home placement were not possible because once again even extremely frail persons (whether in the treatment or control group) with unmet service needs were able to avoid nursing home placement. Many of the most frail elders relied on existing community services and informal caregivers due to their deeply held aversion to nursing home placement.

A more comprehensive model than channeling is the social/health maintenance organization (SHMO), which has been in development since 1980 and is now being tested at four sites: Kaiser Permanente in Portland, Seniors Plus in Minneapolis, SCAN in Long Beach, and Elder Plan in Brooklyn (Leutz et al., 1985). The SHMO is similar to the HMO in its emphasis on capitation rather than fee for service, but it also combines acute care and long-term care services, which are financed through Medicare and Medicaid waivers. Moreover, the SHMO will actually deliver a complete package of services to elderly enrollees, versus the more typical referral thrust of channeling and other case management programs. The SHMO Medicare and Medicaid waivers were authorized through a provision of the Deficit Reduction Act of 1984.

The SHMO was originally conceived and developed by investigators at Brandeis University, with primary evaluation of the four programs in divergent milieu conducted by the Aging Health Policy Center at the University of California in San Francisco. One of the major criteria for success will be financial solvency. The financial viability of SHMOs will be based on two events: (1) enrollment that includes a sufficiently large number of members who will not need services in a given year and (2) case managers who access the least intensive care that is appropriate for a given individual. Eventually the Health Care Financing Administration will shift full financial responsibility to the SHMO, which will depend on the collection of Medicare reimbursements, additional enrollee premiums, and specific copayments for its survival.

Another foray into acute care *and* community long-term care (albeit small and tentative in the latter regard) is the Catastrophic Protection Act. The most publicized accomplishment of this proposed legislation is that no one will pay more than $2,000 out of pocket for hospital care. Thus, after a deductible is met, Medicare shifts from being a limited protection plan to an unlimited one. Unfortunately, less than one half of 1% of Medicare's 32 million beneficiaries will benefit from such a plan. The vast majority are struggling with long-term care needs, most of which are in the community.

In response to this need the legislation does address community long-term care issues as well. Provisions of the act allow small improvements in home health care, add prescription drug coverage after a substantial annual deductible is met, improve protection of assets and income of the spouse of a nursing home resident, require the state to pay cost-sharing components of Medicare for all beneficiaries under the poverty line, and add a small respite provision. These additional benefits will be financed through increased Part B Medicare premiums and, for those higher income recipients, an income-related supplemental premium as part of the federal income tax. This financing method would be the first income-based financing method to pay for Medicare benefits and the first treatment of in-kind benefits as taxable income. Also, while long-term care benefits are addressed in a token way, Medicare benefits will for the first time include nonmedical services of use to persons in the home.

ADULT DAY CARE

In the absence of both a national long-term care policy and widespread funding sources, adult day care centers in the United States still manage to proliferate (Mace & Rabins, 1984). From none in 1970, adult day care sites expanded to 250+ in 1978, to 600+ in 1980, and to 1400+ in 1987.

The objective of adult day care is to provide a protective community setting for those unable to remain unsupervised during the day in their own homes and who do not have the family or other informal caregiving support during these daylight hours. The variety of adult day care services can range from mere supervision to include nutrition, health and social services, therapeutic and recreational activities, counseling, self-care training, and transportation to and from the site.

Typical candidates for adult day care are those who have mobility problems, have a tendency to wander, require assistance with toileting, are unable to adhere to a medication schedule, or are confused. Those centers accommodating a high percentage of clients with dementia will be more limited in the number of clients they can manage per staff person, their staff will need additional training, and there will be an increased need for volunteer help. Pfeiffer et al. (1985) suggest that all staff and volunteers at such centers receive training in the following: coping with memory loss problems; developing crisis intervention strategies with combative patients; improving listening skills; understanding the effects of dementia on family; managing stress; and developing assessment skills and intervention strategies such as remotivation therapy, reality orientation, and sensory deprivation rehabilitation.

Day care centers are most likely to be affiliated with nursing homes, community mental health centers, state psychiatric hospitals, churches, religious organizations, or senior centers. The most likely sources of funding are client fees, private endowment, Medicaid reimbursement, Social Services Block Grant, and Older American Act funds (Mace & Rabins, 1984).

From a cost containment perspective, adult day care is a viable publicly supported option if additional public funds are not needed for supervision during the evenings and weekends. Gurewitsch (1983) argues that many older persons live with a working caregiver and the adult day care site allows the caregiver to continue working during traditional work hours. Thus, public support for a more expensive setting, typically a nursing home, can be avoided.

During the past 5 years state and federal funding has increased for adult day care centers. By 1986, for instance, 15 states were providing Medicaid reimbursement, partially stimulated by Medicaid waivers authorized under Section 2176 of the 1981 Omnibus Budget Reconciliation Act. On the other hand, private sector businesses and insurance companies continue to resist employee or consumer coverage for adult day care benefits. Under 5% of the adult day care sites, for example, receive reimbursement from private insurance companies.

There are some interesting exceptions to the private sector's resistance to reimbursement of adult day care. A project funded by the Administration on Aging and conducted by the National Association of Area Agencies on Aging, for instance, is examining the impact that Wang Laboratories in Massachusetts is having on employees by contracting with adult day care centers to provide respite for their employee-caregivers. The Travelers Company in Hartford, Connecticut, and Group Health Cooperative in Puget Sound, Washington, are also including coverage for adult day care as a new benefit for employees.

The promise of adult day care may be realized through the self-interest of the large contingency of working baby boomers who are just now entering the peak adult child caregiving ages of the 40s and 50s. These baby boom activists are likely to advocate for employee caregiving benefits. If these benefits are not forthcoming through employers, another alternative is Medicare reimbursement for adult day care. Plans that involved additional government reimbursements, however, have limited potential in the era of cost containment, unless researchers can document them as cost-effective alternatives to other publicly funded programs.

Other barriers to day care that need to be addressed are the public's lack of knowledge of available facilities, the limited accessibility of some sites, the need to foster referrals from provider agencies, the hesitancy of family members to entrust the care of the older person, and the need for additional funding sources that could assist families with modest means as well as those that are destitute. In the face of these challenges, 70% to 80% of adult day care centers have operated under capacity (Mace & Rabins, 1984).

An alternative to adult day care in the community is short-term respite in an institutional setting. This type of respite can target needs other than those of a working caregiver needing daytime relief. Institutional respite is most suited to those caregivers who want relief for 24 hours, a weekend, or several days on end. Typically, it takes place in a nursing home, though it can be applied to licensed residential facilities, foster homes, or hospitals. To provide short-term respite, an institution would need to be able to operate on short notice, streamline its admission procedures, and train staff to minimize the confusion associated with repeated relocations.

LONG-TERM CARE INSURANCE

The potential for establishing long-term care insurance plans is limited by the generally shared belief among underwriters that the long-term care population constitutes an unpredictable insurance risk. Even the "pooled risk" concept, which aims for greater predictability through a larger population pool that includes low-risk users as well as high-risk users, may not apply very well to the long-term care population. This is because even the larger population of potential long-term care users is likely to have a pent-up demand for community- or institutional-based long-term care services. In other words, a sizable but uncertain number of persons have been making do without formal services that are for them unavailable, unaffordable, or, in the case of nursing homes, unacceptable. Given the uncertainty of how widespread the demand for long-term care actually is, the insurer's response is likely to be to screen out those people who are the most vulnerable: low-income persons who cannot share costs, those afflicted with Alzheimer's disease, those with preexisting conditions, and so forth.

The inability to predict service need is one factor that dampens enthusiasm in the private sector toward long-term care insurance. Another factor is that the younger, healthier population in the work force is difficult to attract into a pooled risk system. Many people in the working population in their 30s, 40s, 50s, and even 60s, ignore long-range health care planning. The lack of foresight among many employees is typically matched by the lack of enthusiasm among employers toward expanding health benefits. When the long-term care insurance option is made available to employees the benefit involves high premiums (more than double the amount of medi-gap premiums), high deductibles, and limits on coverage—especially for home care services.

An analysis of 31 long-term care policies reveals how limited private long-term care coverage really is. Wiener and associates (1987) report that low option plans have long deductible periods, coverage as short as 1 year, and reimbursement that averages as low as $40 a day. This low option plan averages $318 in premium costs for persons age 65 and $728 for persons age 79. (High option plans average $1,496 for persons age 79.) In contrast, medi-gap premiums range from $234 to $473 according to a six-state survey.

A government sponsored long-term care insurance program, perhaps a

Medicare Part C option, could avoid the adverse selection problem faced by private insurance companies. Distributing the cost of insurance over the entire population would maximize the pooled risk, thereby maximizing coverage and keeping individual costs down. Moreover, in the year 2010, when the baby boomers begin to need long-term care assistance, substantial financial services would have accumulated ahead of time.

If a Medicare Part C option becomes a reality, a difficult decision has to be made—how much of the benefits should be financed through user premiums versus how much through general tax revenues. As has happened with Medicare Part B, when the entitlement mentality takes hold of the public there is increasing pressure to keep premiums down and to shift financing to general revenue. In the era of cost containment, however, individual premiums are encouraged over options that raise taxes. Thus, Representative Claude Pepper (D-FL) proposed the Long Term Home Care Bill in 1987 (H.R. 3436), which was to be financed by removal of the cap on income subject to the Medicare part of the payroll tax (1.45% of $45,000 in 1988).

As Wiener and colleagues (1987) suggest, a two-tiered approach similar to Social Security and private pensions may be forthcoming. The first tier could be an expanded public insurance program that includes long-term care to provide a modest degree of protection for everyone. This could be financed, as Pepper suggests, through a payroll tax shared by employees and employers without the salary cap on the existing Medicare program. The second tier, which could be financed through private insurance companies, the government, or a combination of the two, would offer a more expanded level of coverage for those able to pay a premium along with other out-of-pocket costs.

SUPPORTIVE HOUSING

For older persons who have minor problems but who are still living independently, there is a wide variety of housing options that could be appropriate. *Government subsidized housing for the elderly,* for instance, refers to 1.5 million housing units occupied by the elderly, with rents that are adjusted to the low-income resident's net income. Typically, services such as meals, heavy housekeeping, recreation, and access to a nurse are available to tenants. Residents must qualify by having assets and an annual income below a certain level, along with having a sufficient degree of autonomy. Federally subsidized congregate housing facilities were a low priority under the Reagan administration, and the availability of congregate housing in the future may depend on the willingness of nonprofit organizations to sponsor them.

Since 60% of the elderly own homes with no mortgage remaining, a *life care facility* can meet the need of a more affluent segment of the older adult population. For those who are able to sell their homes at a sufficient profit to afford the large initial payment (typically $60,000 to $100,000) and ongoing monthly fees ($1,000 or more), the life care facility will provide a wide variety of medical and nursing services, residential support services, and social activities. If a resident is transferred to a long-term care facility, there is a guarantee of a return to the life care facility if health should permit. In 1981 there were 100,000 residents in about 300 life care facilities (U.S. Senate Special Committee on Aging, 1986).

Congregate housing and life care facilities share an age-segregated approach to the home environment. Rosow's (1967) research on apartment buildings in Cleveland and Detroit suggests that such age-segregated housing can be beneficial to mental and physical health. From a mental health view, the older resident can avoid the stigma of growing older in the larger society. Instead, residents can enhance their self-esteem through identifying with similar life circumstances among neighbors and increasing interaction with neighbors and friends. From a physical health perspective, the congregate facility is likely to include a variety of safety features that are appropriate for older adults that are not commonly available in age-integrated environments.

Conversely, the insulation of age-segregated housing from the larger society deprives both the older and the younger generation of the complementarity of intergenerational living. The old provide the young with a continuity to the past and the wisdom they have gathered through experience; the young provide the old with enthusiasm, vitality, and eagerness to explore new ideas. Nationwide, 78% of older Americans prefer to live in a neighborhood with all ages, and a surprising 33% of those who already live in an age-segregated housing site prefer a building with all age groups (American Association of Retired Persons, 1988).

In addition, Carp (1976) and Sheehan (1986) reported that age-segregated housing may only be beneficial to some tenants and not others. High levels of social interaction and support among tenants in age-segregated housing, for instance, may be limited to those who are the most healthy. Through interviews with housing authorities and older tenants, Sheehan (1986) found that increased frailty is associated with increased isolation. At a time when support is needed the most, it may be available the least.

Frail residents report a reluctance to burden others, especially since they are not in a position to reciprocate. Even during periods of maximum vulnerability, such as a recent discharge from a hospital, frail residents are reluctant to seek help from neighbors. The healthier neighbors, in turn, report that family and formal service agencies are supposed to help with frail elders, not neighbors. The healthy residents noted their limited energy level and doubted their capacity to be an adequate source of help for the substantially impaired neighbor (Sheehan, 1986).

A demonstration program to encourage healthy, older tenant volunteers to help frail neighbors in housing for the elderly was launched in 1987. This demonstration project, funded by the Administration on Aging, identifies tenants who need help with personal care or instrumental activities and matches them with helpers willing to assist in specific areas of need (Gutkin, 1987). Given shrinking and dispersed family units and the limits on formal services in this era of cost containment, the congregate living facility can be an important milieu for assisting the frail elder.

Two supportive housing options that are not necessarily age segregated are house sharing and board and care homes. *House sharing* involves unrelated people living together. Benefits from such housing can include companionship, financial savings, care for a frail person, or assistance around the house. One popular form of exchange initiated by older persons who own their homes is the lowering of rents to young adults with limited incomes in exchange for services rendered: yard work, errands, household chores, and so on.

The two ways in which house sharing differs from the age-old practice of "taking in a boarder" are (1) the use of matching programs, which are proliferating around the country and are attempting to increase the chances of locating compatible persons and (2) the development of creative ways to share financial and daily living responsibilities. Potential house sharers must be cognizant of zoning laws that permit unrelated people to share a home and the impact that house sharing may have on taxes, supplementary security income, and food stamp benefits.

The other supportive housing option that might foster intergenerational living is the *board and care home* (also referred to as the adult foster care home, domiciliary care home, sheltered care facility, or halfway house). Board and care homes provide room, board, utilities, and supervision. Sometimes they also provide social, recreational, and spiritual activities; housekeeping and laundry services; and assistance with obtaining medication or supervision of its usage. In many states, however, licensing for safety and health is not required, and the quality of such homes varies greatly. Even with licensing, board and care facilities have been known to vary tremendously regarding cleanliness, privacy, security, freedom to bring one's own furnishings, and the scope of services or activities available on the premises. Most of the 30,000+ board and care homes are family owned and operated, with half of the estimated 370,000 residents age 65 or older (Reichstein & Bergofsky, 1983).

The most desirable option for most people seeking supportive housing is to receive needed services *in the home*. Remaining in the comfort and security of one's own home gives one a sense of control and peace of mind. In addition to maintaining a familiar home environment, one can maintain social involvement with neighbors, community organizations, and long-time employees of neighborhood commercial establishments. Departure to another home often means leaving valued personal possessions as well as social contacts.

The most sought after support services in the home are personal care (dressing, bathing, etc.) and chore services (shopping, meal preparation, light housekeeping, etc.) provided by home health aides and homemakers. The most frequently used health care professionals are nurses, physical and occupational therapists, speech and hearing therapists, social workers, and nutritionists. Finding the right combination of affordable professionals and services typically requires agency help, whether it is through a private/nonprofit or profit-making agency, a hospital-based department, or a public health department.

Typically the first step in establishing a supportive care plan for the home is through a physician. If skilled services are reimbursable through Medicare, Medicaid, Title III of the Older Americans Act, the Social Services Block Grant, or private insurance plans, the physician's approval is necessary for meeting eligibility requirements. Given that long-term care knowledge must be self-taught rather than learned in medical school, it is wise to supplement the physician's knowledge base with additional sources of information. Other valuable resource persons are personnel from area agencies on aging, social service/public health/Social Security administration departments, churches/synagogues, hospital discharge planners, and nursing home social workers. If necessary, the yellow pages (or silver pages published by Southwestern Bell Media in St. Louis) can reveal important services and resources in the local area.

Financing home support is typically borne by the individual. Medicare, for instance, does not provide personal care or chore services and provides only limited home health care. Since Medicare's statutory language is vague in defining the terms *intermittent care, skilled care,* and *homebound,* the regional fiscal intermediaries are inconsistent with approving eligibility for Medicare reimbursement. Qualifying for Medicaid reimbursement is difficult because of eligibility limits on monthly income and assets (property value, savings accounts, etc.). Moreover, eligibility and scope of coverage vary by state since each state is responsible for its own Medicaid program. Thus, many agencies do not accept Medicaid patients because the actual cost of care exceeds that which the state Medicaid program will reimburse.

Another source of financing home care is a private insurance policy. Many such policies have recently included home health care in their coverage, but with substantial limitations. Also veterans may qualify for home care assistance by contacting the nearest Veterans Administration hospital. An increasing number of VA home health care programs, however, are restricted to service-connected disabilities. Finally, religious, fraternal, civic, and neighborhood organizations offer home health care assistance to those in need.

A final source of financing home care support is home equity conversion, a financial plan that allows homeowners to borrow against the equity in their homes with repayment postponed into the future—preferably after death with proceeds from the sale of the home. Since 70% of all elderly persons own their own home, including two thirds of low-income aged persons, this plan could allow many elders the lifetime use of their home (Jacobs, 1985). A nationwide survey revealed that one fourth of persons age 60 and over would consider the home equity conversion option (American Association of Retired Persons, 1988). About 100 home equity conversions had taken place by 1984 (Weinrobe, 1984). In 1987 the Connecticut State Housing Authority became one of the first public agencies to help elderly homeowners finance long-term care through a home equity conversion. The $45 million program is coordinated through the Connecticut Department on Aging.

The most valuable home care resource, of course, is the *informal caregiver,* typically a family member. More than any other resource person, it is the informal caregiver who provides the necessary housecleaning, meal preparation, grocery shopping, laundry services, medication supervision, personal hygiene assistance, and so forth. The informal caregiver will endure with caregiving responsibilities more successfully if given proper training (see list of caregiving books in Appendix B) and adequate respite. Without these sources of support primary caregivers are more vulnerable to committing psychologically abusive acts or neglect. Given the importance of the informal caregiver, Coward (1983) calls for studies that will predict those circumstances that are likely to lead to caregiving abuse.

HOSPICE

Medieval travelers on difficult journeys stopped for rest at wayside shelters called hospices. Modern-day travelers, so to speak, on their way from this life to the next state of being (or nonbeing) are also stopping at hospices for rest. Hospices for terminally ill persons and their family caregivers began at St. Christopher's in London, England in 1967. Since the first American hospice, Connecticut Hospice, Inc., in New Haven, was founded in 1974, more than 1,000 have opened and more than 100,000 persons are being served annually.

The hospice movement has two main goals. First, it is necessary to relieve or eliminate symptoms of pain and discomfort for patients who, for the most part, have a prognosis of 6 months or less to live. Second, it is essential to affirm life through physical, emotional, social, and spiritual support for the dying person and the family. Hospice care is a team effort and includes the patient, the family, friends, volunteers, physicians, nurses, social workers, clergy, and bereavement counselors. Hospices can be based in hospitals, nursing homes, or homes, through a combination of inpatient and home care services.

The hospice may not be for everyone. To some people it may be tainted by euthanasia or the idea that hospices simply help people die. To an increasing number of persons, however, the hospice is a means for helping people live their remaining months in a more comfortable environment than one with an institutional decor and an abundance of bureaucratic regulations. Hospices, even if they are hospital based, try to maximize the comforts of home and to minimize unnecessary constraints in the environment. There are few rules regarding decorating one's room, visiting hours, meal schedules, use of alcohol, pets, special foods, and use of pain control strategies.

Medicare began covering hospice care in 1983. Reimbursement (in 1987) is limited to 210 days of care, and the reimbursement level seldom covers the actual costs of hospice care. There are alternatives to federally subsidized hospice care. In 1986 Congress considered a bill to allow states to add a hospice benefit to their Medicaid programs (Hospice benefits, 1985). Also the number of private insurance plans offering hospice benefits continues to increase. More than half of the Fortune 500 companies, for instance, have added hospice coverage to their employees' insurance plan (Hospice benefits, 1985). This is not a surprising trend, given the number of studies that demonstrate that inpatient hospice care saves more than 50% of the costs incurred through traditional hospital care and that home-based hospice care can reap even more savings. In contrast to the hospice approach, one study reported that the 6% of Medicare beneficiaries who died in 1978 accounted for 28% of Medicare expenditures over a 2-year period (Lubitz & Prihoda, 1984).

At the present time about two thirds of hospice patients are over the age of 65, and this proportion will increase as the proportion of elderly in the population increases (Butterfield-Picard & Magno, 1982). A major problem with hospice users who are elderly is that a home-based support system is frequently nonexistent or inadequate. Many spouses and adult children in their 60s and 70s are unable to bear the exhausting burden of primary caregiving with the terminally ill. To meet the challenge of providing hospice care for elderly persons without adequate primary care, hospice programs may be more dependent on inpatient care where adequate support and supervision is available. Due to the greater costs associated with inpatient hospice care, however, Medicare regulations limit the inpatient days that hospice programs will be reimbursed in comparison to home care days. Thus, there is additional need for volunteers to help meet the needs of the terminally ill elderly with inadequate support (Lupu, 1984–1985).

II

COST–CONSCIOUS COMMUNITY CARE

4

INFORMAL CAREGIVING

To provide appropriate health care for an aging society, policymakers must contend with a paradox. On the one hand, the emotional, financial, and physical costs of maintaining older persons at home or in the community rest primarily with the family. On the other hand, social and health policies ignore or penalize family members caring for frail older relatives at home. This paradox is heading toward crisis proportions as the nation's supply of frail elderly living at home escalates and the society's stock of family caregivers diminishes and copes with increasing demands (for women) in the work sector.

This chapter examines the centrality of home care, family caregiving, and community volunteer caregiving in the long-term care system of today, as well as the caregiver's need for information, support, and respite in providing care for older persons at home.

HOME CARE

Home care can be broadly defined as a range of services in the home setting in which there is typically significant involvement of family, friends, or neighbors in the caregiving process. Home care services range from telephone calls by family or friends for checking-up purposes to nursing and rehabilitative services provided by skilled professionals.

Eighty percent of the home care assistance needed by frail elders is provided by informal caregivers: family members, friends, neighbors, and volunteers (Doty, 1984; Nelson, 1982; Rabin & Stockton, 1987). Spousal (36%) and child (32%) support account for much of this assistance, and other relatives contribute significantly as well (22%) (Rabin & Stockton, 1987).

The vast majority of federal funding for home care, however, is targeted to medical personnel. In 1980 the medically oriented Medicare program accounted for 81% of publicly funded home care. Medicare recipients eligible for home care must be homebound, in need of skilled care under a physician-directed plan, and capable of making progress toward normalcy through rehabilitative efforts.

The first federal program (in 1960) to provide home care assistance for the aged did reimburse eligible persons for nonmedical chronic care for the functionally disabled at home. Since then, other federally funded programs such as Section 2176 of Title XIX of the Social Security Act (the Medicaid waiver program), Title XX program of the Social Security Act (Social Services Block Grant), Title III of the Older Americans Act (supportive services), and certain Veterans Administration programs have included nonmedical services in the home. In general, though, the trend toward the "medical model," or federal reimbursement for skilled care, has become the general policy.

The Omnibus Reconciliation Act of 1980, however, has been an attempt to liberalize home care benefits under the Medicare and Medicaid programs. Proprietary agencies, for instance, could join nonprofit home health care agencies in the provision of home care services. Also, the limits on the number of visits, the prior hospitalization requirement, and the Medicare Part B deductible were eliminated. Finally, federal guidelines allowed the states greater flexibility in the provision of nonmedical home care services.

Due to the increased number of shortened hospital stays as a consequence of Medicare's prospective payment system, home health care became the fastest growing component of Medicare in 1985 with expenditures of $2.3 billion. Because of budget constraints, however, severe limits on these services were imposed at the state level. These limits included the number of home visits allowed, continuation of physician supervision, and a narrow range of eligible services.

By 1984 18 states had implemented a prospective payment system for home health services, which frequently discouraged home health agencies from even participating in the reimbursement system. These cost limits on home health care services reduced the amount an agency could charge for a unit of service at a time when more acutely ill patients were leaving hospitals and needing more intensive (expensive) home health care services. Prospective payment systems in effect forced agencies to consider case-mix policies, that is, to seek primarily patients who do not require more costly home health care services.

To cope with rising home care costs at the federal level, the Health Care Financing Administration implemented two cost containment initiatives in 1985. First, a cost limit on allowable charges (based on previous average home visit costs) was set, regardless of actual cost of service. The second policy was to increase claim denials, which jeopardized the home health agency's waiver of liability; that is, an exemption for payment of claim denials less than 2.5% of visits billed per quarter. The waiver of liability was granted to home health agencies by fiscal intermediaries to permit a steady cash flow and to allow for budgetary planning. This waiver has been essential for smaller agencies with limited cash reserves. Despite the necessity of a waiver, a survey of 36 home health agencies in New Jersey in 1985 revealed that "39% reported loss of waiver of liability in the last year, and 72% reported an increase in denials over the past six months" (Taylor, 1986).

Thus, the cost containment revolution in the hospitals has major implications for home care. Patients are more likely to be discharged to the home with a greater degree of frailty, but at the same time home health care agencies must grapple with new cost containment initiatives designed to curtail medical expenses outside of the hospital. The issue of allowing nonmedical, chronic care reimbursement for older persons functioning in a reasonably stable manner is, for obvious cost reasons, addressed only periodically and tentatively by federal officials. At the same time, however, the severity of medical problems at home continues to increase, along with the family caregiving strain (Johnson & Catalano, 1983).

Access to nursing home care by hospital patients who are being discharged earlier is increasingly constrained in many states as well. As nursing homes continue to seek patients with limited nursing care requirements (not to mention those who are private pay as well), long-term care alternatives for many family caregivers will be severely curtailed.

FAMILY CAREGIVING

Caregiving refers to the range of interpersonal activities that is provided by family, friends, neighbors, and volunteers to assist an individual with his or her physical, psychological, and social needs (Scott & Roberto, 1985). Caregiving activities refer to supervision or checking-up activities, material guidance or help, personal care, companionship or comfort, encouragement, and information (Pearson, 1982). Informal caregiving is important because the vast majority of older Americans and their family members prefer living at home, where there is maximum personal choice, privacy, and dignity. Unlike institutional living, there are few restrictions imposed by others governing personal possessions, social interaction, eating schedules, choice of interior decoration, and so forth. In short, living at home provides the maximum amount of self-determination.

While family caregiving to older adults has been part of the American tradition since the birth of the nation, the scope of this responsibility has increased in recent years. One major factor has been that the percentage of persons over age 65 has tripled during the 20th century. Even more important, the

80 and over population, which is most susceptible to becoming care recipients, has become the nation's fastest growing age group. Currently the mean age of older care recipients is 77.7 (Stone, 1986), but it is expected to rise along with the population's mean age.

Several million Americans provide help to an older relative on any given day, with more than 2 million providing substantial assistance to a frail older person (Stone, 1986). One third of the caregivers are over age 65 themselves and are at the age when they too can become physically vulnerable. In addition to age, gender is an important caregiving factor. Women not only constitute three out of four caregivers, they are more likely to provide difficult types of assistance such as personal care. Also, among caregiving daughters over half are grappling with job issues such as cutting back on work hours, rearranging schedules, taking time off without pay to fulfill caregiving duties, or having to resign their jobs to become full-time caregivers. Ironically, many caregiving women outlive their husbands and, since three out of four nursing home residents are women, they wind up receiving impersonal caregiving in nursing homes.

The need for caregiving support at home increases with age to compensate for cumulative physical, psychological, economical, and social losses (Scott & Roberto, 1985). While cumulative losses typically require ongoing emotional support for low-stress situations (Cohen et al., 1985), a person's vulnerability to crisis increases with age as well. Thus, the support network must be enlarged, or the services to be performed must expand, to include additional emotional support, physical assistance and material aid (Cohen et al., 1985; Preston & Mansfield, 1984; Stephens & Bernstein, 1984). If expansion of support cannot occur during these crises, the emotional strain can build and lead to the dissolution of the informal caregiving network (Johnson & Catalano, 1983).

Both ongoing low-stress support and crisis-oriented support will be harder to come by due to social and demographic trends:

> *(a) as the number of frail elderly increases dramatically, the number of adult children as care givers will decrease, primarily due to declining birth rates and increasing residential mobility; (b) as women continue to provide 70–75% of all informal care giving in the community, competing demands on their time also increase, especially due to labor force participation and heading of single-parent households; and (c) as the "aging of the aged" occurs it is accompanied by the aging of adult children and spousal care givers, thus increasing everyone's physical vulnerability. (Haber, 1986b)**

*From Haber, D. In-home and community-based long-term care services: A review of recent AOA projects involving self-determination. *Journal of Applied Gerontology, 5*(1), 37–50. Copyright 1986 by Sage Publications, Inc. Reprinted with permission.

Complicating the fact that family size is shrinking is the trend over the past 4 decades of women entering the work force in increasing numbers. Moreover, this trend of taking on an economic role in the family has not preempted the woman's primary caregiving role. Thus, women are being asked to give up both the flexibility of schedule and the easy access to an impaired older relative that the homemaker role affords (Brody et al., 1983). To cope with these dual responsibilities, women employee/caregivers are adhering to rigid schedules and giving up much of their free time (Cantor, 1983; Horowitz et al., 1983; Lang & Brody, 1983). The strain becomes especially severe for the older working woman who typically cares for a very old, especially frail, parent (Brody, 1985). Some of these women are forced to reduce working hours or quit work altogether.

A study of adult daughter caregivers to elderly widowed women in Philadelphia documents that working-caregiving daughters do not give fewer hours to their caregiving responsibilities than nonworking daughters (Brody & Schoonover, 1986). Perhaps the major concession to the work-caregiving conflict is the greater willingness of the caregiver to share personal care and meal preparation with a paid worker. Otherwise, housework, laundry, transportation, shopping, money management, and other caregiving services are similar to those of the nonworking caregiving daughter (Brody & Schoonover, 1986).

The issue of working caregiving daughters will become even more salient as the trend toward more working women continues. Between 1940 and 1979 the percentage of working married women rose from 11% to almost 56%. Among the most probable group of caregivers, women age 45 to 54, 60% are in the labor force (Brody, 1981). Among those age 55 to 64, 42% work (U.S. Bureau of Labor Statistics, 1984). So far the rising proportions of working caregiving daughters has not meant abandonment of family members. However, the changing role of the female caregiver who works and what types of assistance she will need will be a very important research topic for the next few decades.

The myth that the family has abandoned its caregiving responsibilities to elderly members has been thoroughly discredited by researchers. Shanas (1979) has documented a high incidence of family support to impaired elderly, and studies report that family members are crucial for allowing the elderly to remain at home (Brody et al., 1978). As mentioned, for every severely disabled elderly person in an institution, at least two equally impaired older people live with and are cared for by family members (Brody et al., 1978; Laurie, 1978).

Family loyalty can be so intense, however, it can lead to elderly abuse in times of health care crisis. Some children, regardless of circumstances, are unable to relinquish approval-seeking from their parent or the guilt of having been supported during dependency without an opportunity for reciprocity (Brody, 1985). A study (Johnson & Catalano, 1983) of more than 100 elderly discharged from hospitals reported that the potential for family abuse increases along with the increased dependency of elderly family members. The emphasis on maintaining family caregiving in times of stress and the lack of acceptable alternatives can drive family members beyond their capacity to manage normal activities.

The guilt feeling that pushes adult children to support their parents beyond their capacity is illustrated by the following anecdote. A physician summarized a case presentation he made to a class of graduate nurses (Ruskin, 1983). Among the characteristics of his patient, who was a "white female who appeared her reported age," were babbling incoherently; disorientation regarding time, place, and person; disregard of physical appearance; being edentulous and incontinent; inability to feed, bathe, or clothe herself; erratic sleep pattern; and agitation without apparent cause. After obtaining consistently negative reactions to being responsible for this patient's care from the student nurses, the physician reported that, on the contrary, he enjoyed taking care of his 6-month-old daughter. He concluded, "We need to change our perspective. The aged patient is just as lovable as the child."

Perhaps adult children do find their very old parents as lovable as their own children. They certainly do not find them as "careable." The adult caregiver has increasing independence to look forward to in caring for an infant but decreasing independence in caring for a parent. Sometimes this dependency is characterized by decreasing physical ability, mental ability, and 'lovability' in the parent as well. Since one third of the caregivers are also age 65 or over and a comparable percentage are near poor or poor and perceive their own health status as fair or poor (Stone et al., 1986), dwindling physical, financial, and emotional resources become a challenge as well.

While family abandonment or abuse remains rare, the stress of family caregiving is likely to increase over the next few decades because of the shrinking and dispersing family network. Future cohorts of elderly will have fewer family supports to depend on due to declining birthrates. Within the 5-year period from 1975 to 1980 alone, for instance, the average family size dropped from 3.4 to 3.1 (Callahan et al., 1980).

Geographical mobility is also a factor, as indicated by a national survey that reported that more than one in four children had an elderly parent who lived more than 150 miles away from them (Moss et al., 1985). It is not surprising, therefore, that a study of newspaper obituary columns in a midwestern city reported that 25% of those age 65 years and older at the time of death had no surviving children or siblings residing nearby to provide regular direct assistance (Hays, 1984). Perhaps even more important to note about this study is that less than half had that most important human resource—a daughter—residing within 50 miles of them.

Families differ in many ways. Without question, however, the most significant variation in terms of caregiving is the presence of a daughter or a daughter-in-law. A study of nine different federally funded model projects revealed that

83% of all the caregivers were women (Dichter et al., 1981; Hofer, 1980). Another study of New York City caregivers (Horowitz, 1985) examined the difference between sons and daughters as caregivers. First, the researchers found that 76% of the children giving care were daughters. Second, among the 24% who were caregiving sons, many became caregivers by default; that is, they were members of families without daughters or they were the only geographically accessible child.

Given the preponderance of women as informal caregivers, wives and daughters determine the strength of most caregiving networks (Brody, 1981, 1985; Johnson & Catalano, 1983). Daughters are three times more likely than sons to share their households with a dependent elderly parent (Brody & Shoonover, 1986). Women place more emphasis on personal relationships (Gilligan, 1982), have stronger emotional ties to families of origin (Horowitz, 1985), and have stronger social support systems than men (Lowenthal et al., 1975). The overwhelming importance of daughters and wives as the primary caregivers to impaired elders holds true for other countries as well (Kendig & Rowland, 1983).

There are many other interesting variations in family caregiving characteristics that may offer insight into the unique ways that families can—or cannot—cope and obtain resources. Race, for instance, may prove to be an interesting variable to examine. Bengtson (1979), Cantor (1979b), and Taylor (1985) report that elderly blacks give more child rearing assistance, including taking grandchildren, nieces, and nephews into their home, than do elderly whites. On the other hand, adult black children profess less support of family caregiving norms than do whites, perhaps because they have less monetary resources and time with which to accomplish caregiving tasks if called on to do so (Sauer & Seelbach, 1983). Hispanic adult children may provide more support to their elders, even with socioeconomic and health factors controlled (Rosenthal, 1986). At the present time, though, racial comparisons generally tend to reveal more about socioeconomic differences than they do about racial differences (Cantor, 1979b; Jackson, 1980; Mindell et al., 1986; Mitchell & Register, 1984; Rosenthal, 1986; Rubenstein, 1971).

Shifting the focus to socioeconomic differences reveals that low socioeconomic status is associated with more instrumental caregiving, probably because paid alternatives are not available (Rosenthal, 1986). Higher socioeconomic status is associated with more emotional support and the endorsement of family caregiving norms (Sauer & Seelbach, 1983; Weihl, 1983)—once again because there may be more time to help out or more resources with which to pay for the basic tasks of daily assistance.

Other interesting pathways to caregiving insight may come through the study of ethnic factors, that is, shared cultural beliefs and values that guide the behavior of families (Rosenthal, 1986; urban-rural or regional differences (Taylor, 1985); the age of caregivers, which is associated with increased risk of disability or morbidity and the dissolution of the caregiving household (Fitting et al., 1986; Soldo & Myllyluoma, 1983); and family intactness.

Regarding intactness, almost half of all families do not qualify as being "intact," when you add single adults to the ranks of widowed, separated, divorced, and remarried adults (Sussman, 1976). Intactness is important when you consider that disrupted families have greater potential for conflict with former spouses and friends, in-laws, separated children, and other family members. A study of adult children who had experienced marital disruption reported that this event interfered with their ability to help elderly parents over age 60 (Cicirelli, 1983).

Since most older women are widowed, widowhood may constitute the most important example of marital disruption. Studies have shown that some elderly widows have a greater diversity of caregiving providers than married older people because they have been motived to cultivate involvements with extended kin, friends, and neighbors (Brody & Schoonover, 1986; Cantor, 1979a; Johnson & Catalano, 1983; O'Brien & Wagner, 1980). One study, however, reported that childless widows, despite their apparent greater needs, did not receive significantly more support than widows with children (O'Bryant, 1985). Childless widows may have been more career or couple oriented and did not have the primary resources—children—that are used to meet neighbors and to establish neighborhood support networks.

COMMUNITY VOLUNTEER NETWORKS

The wide variety of friends, neighbors, and volunteer networks that impact on so many persons has been referred to as a "massive unregulated social welfare system [which] exists naturally [and] provides more services, security and hope for the future than all our agency help together" (Coe et al., 1984). The composition of this informal network is going to change in the upcoming decades. As the birthrate declines and family members continue to disperse, neighbors, friends, and volunteers will become an increasingly vital thrust to this unregulated welfare system. Already there is evidence that interaction with the neighborhood support system is just as important to maintaining independence among the impaired elderly as interaction with the family network (Coe et al., 1984).

Most community helpers, whether they are friends or neighbors, initiate their own efforts outside of any organized program. *Natural neighbors,* a term coined by Collins and Pancoast (1976), refers to people who are prompted by empathy or a desire to help others. While the assistance of natural neighbors is most often in the form of doing errands or checking up on someone, skilled or intensive services to impaired elders are also provided. Many of these natural neighbors began their volunteer work at churches or formal service agencies, with a substantial number being former nurses, social workers, or teachers

(Goodman, 1984). Some natural neighbors have come from large or religiously oriented families or had parents who helped others.

Many natural neighbors have not only accumulated skills over a lifetime of service, they are willing to make substantial commitments to helping others. Rather than gender, income, or educational level being the primary indicator of willingness to volunteer in late life, often it is the life cycle of previous volunteer efforts that best predicts continuation of service (Chambre, 1984; Morgan et al., 1979). Instead of merely looking for retirement roles to substitute for former work and family responsibilities, these volunteers are continuing a lifelong pattern of values and helping activities.

Some neighbors and volunteers may not be as "natural" or as skillful as others, but they are willing to undertake a paraprofessional training program to increase their skills at performing helping services. One model training program at Washington University in Missouri identified and trained 100 older volunteers to be volunteer case managers. The volunteers were trained by professional social workers to coordinate a variety of home- and community-based support services for approximately 800 frail elders in need (Ozawa, 1985). A similar pilot program in Seattle, called Project Access, teaches volunteers to serve as case managers for elderly clients and their families. An evaluation in 1988 will help the American Association of Retired Persons determine if Project Access should be offered nationally.

Paraprofessional training programs reach into all sectors of long-term care. One such program, for example, focuses on instilling advocacy skills needed by ombudsmen for long-term care facilities and home health programs (Zischka & Jones, 1984). Yet another program trained elderly health advocates to plan, review, and evaluate community agencies on their ability to be responsive to the long-term care needs of older persons (Ehrlich, 1983).

Persons who may not have the motivation or time to join a paraprofessional training program for helping others may be willing to assume important outreach services as part of their full-time jobs. A gatekeeper program in Spokane, Washington (Raschko, 1985), for instance, takes advantage of occupations that have access to information about the status of isolated elders who may be unwilling or unable to request formal community services. These occupations consist of apartment managers, postal carriers, meter readers, utility repair men, and others who could act as outreach workers or gatekeepers. Without a substantial additional commitment to their existing job responsibilities, gatekeepers in the Spokane program contributed almost one of every three referrals made to a case management referral program. A national gatekeeper training program is available through the National Association of State Units on Aging (NASUA) that assists a wide variety of community workers in identifying problems of the elderly as they perform their normal job responsibilities and trains them to make referrals to local health and social service agencies (see Appendix B).

A volunteer role that requires neither training nor experience is that of an outreach worker. Volunteers, many of whom are retirees, reach out to neighbors in their community and distribute newsletters and other information about resources that can benefit impaired elders and their caregivers (Pynoos et al., 1984). Minimal training may be required for simple companionship programs or escort services for impaired elderly. Even frail elderly, the handicapped, and others with telephones can perform vital companionship and supervision functions (Pynoos, 1987). Thus, time, motivation, transportation, and range of skills need not prevent volunteers from performing services such as the outreach, companionship, and referral services which are necessary to maintain frail elders in the community.

At the federal level, funded demonstration projects have developed, evaluated, and replicated training programs for informal caregivers. Two of the most widely recognized projects were the As Parents Grow Older model and the Natural Supports Program. The As Parents Grow Older model was developed by the Institute of Gerontology at the University of Michigan and the Child and Family Services of Michigan, Inc., and funded by the Administration on Aging. The six-session program was designed to educate adult children caregivers and to link them to community services and resources. The evaluation revealed that participants did increase their knowledge about the aging process, as well as gain information about community resources. The findings did not show that this program or linkage to other community resources would make the difference between whether caregivers provided services or not. This program has been widely replicated through national dissemination of its manual.

The Natural Supports Program was conducted by the Community Service Society in New York City and also funded by the Administration on Aging. While similar in intent to the As Parents Grow Older model, it targeted a wider variety of ethnic and socioeconomic populations and focused more on neighbors and friends of the chronically ill older persons than on family members. The evaluation revealed that regardless of ethnic and income background, caregivers experience stress in their roles and report benefits from caregiving training programs and support groups.

There are three major federally supported volunteer programs through ACTION: the Senior Companion program, the Foster Grandparent program, and the Retired Senior Volunteer program (RSVP). The Senior Companion program is for low-income persons age 60 and over to provide companionship and care to older adults in need. The senior companion receives a small stipend (below minimum wage) to provide part-time (typically 20 hours a week) support services. By September 1981 there were 80 projects around the country, with 5,280 companions.

The Foster Grandparent program matches low-income persons age 60 and over with mentally, physically, or emotionally handicapped children. Foster grandparents provide companionship and guidance to these children with exceptional needs, especially in such settings as hospitals, centers for the retarded, correctional facilities, and other institutions that serve children. The small stipend and 20-hour-a-week schedule also apply to this program. By September 1981 there were 233 projects and 18,030 older volunteers.

RSVP targets retired or semiretired persons age 60 and over who are willing to serve without any financial compensation. RSVP volunteers perform a wide variety of services in all types of community settings. By 1982 there were more than 700 projects with 260,000 volunteers.

Studies on the three programs consistently report that in addition to providing a positive impact on young and old persons in need, the senior volunteers themselves benefit in terms of mental and physical health (ACTION, 1984, 1985).

Another large-scale volunteer effort by older persons is organized through the American Association of Retired Persons, which has trained and placed several thousand volunteers in hundreds of communities to perform an array of volunteer jobs. The AARP Volunteer Talent Bank provides this service nationwide through computerized matching of volunteer talent and interest with appropriate opportunities to serve. AARP, along with the National Council on the Aging, provides booklets for developing and sustaining volunteer programs (see Appendix B).

5

CONGREGATIONS AND CORPORATIONS

CONGREGATIONAL SUPPORT GROUPS

Eighty-five percent of the assistance received by older Americans is provided by the informal support system of family and friends. The ubiquity of informal caregiving is testimony to societal values that prefer family and community support to reliance on social service agencies or long-term care institutions. It is important, however, that this pervasive informal support system not be taken for granted. Studies show that, if family members and others do not gain access to relevant information, skills, and community resources to assist them in their caregiving roles, they are more likely to succumb to physical, emotional, and financial stresses. These stresses increase their vulnerability and that of their care recipient to higher rates of morbidity, institutionalization, and mortality (Mindel, 1980; Oktay & Volland, 1981; Robinson & Thurnher, 1979).

Additional studies have demonstrated that social service agencies have drawbacks in playing the lead role in providing caregiving educational services. First, many elderly and their caregivers lack knowledge about social service agencies and the services they provide (D.C. Office on Aging, 1978). Second, even when knowledge about services is not a problem, the majority of older caregivers and recipients are unwilling to admit need for, or accept help from, social service agencies (D.C. Office of Aging, 1978; Hawkins & Jacobson, 1980). Third, funding for service agencies is not guaranteed over long periods of time, but caregiving needs are ongoing.

The neighborhood church, synagogue, or mosque, on the other hand, could be an ideal site for providing ongoing assistance to informal caregivers (Cantor

& Mayor, 1978; Dancy, 1977; Haber, 1984a,b; Haugk, 1976; Rosen, 1974). The religious institution is typically a stable force in the community and accessible within the immediate neighborhood. Congregational members share values, beliefs, traditions, cultural bonds, and the trust and respect these engender. Religious leaders have historically played a familiar and trusted role in helping strengthen the family. The building itself typically provides a quiet, private, and ample space for meeting the needs of congregation members. Most important of all, the vast majority of the elderly and their caregivers in this nation attend religious services in the faith of their choice (Gallup, 1977).

Gerontological leaders consider the church and synagogue to be the most important resource for the elderly (Palmore, 1980; Payne, 1986). Older persons, in fact, constitute the largest age group in organized religion (Riessman et al., 1984). More than 80% of Americans past age 65 claim their religious faith is the most important influence in their lives (Moberg, 1983). Most important, when help is needed for a problem the religious institution is the most sought after resource (Tobin & Ellor, 1983).

There are three potential barriers, however, to religious congregations helping members acquire the necessary skills, knowledge, and resources for their informal caregiving role. First, the church, synagogue, or mosque is sometimes narrowly defined as a place for ministering only to spiritual needs. These views can be held by social service agency staff or congregation members themselves (Tobin, 1982). Second, the religious institution lacks an organized system for providing services outside of pastoral counseling and visiting the homebound (Tobin, 1982). Third, religious leaders tend not to have gerontological training. A study of Milwaukee clergy, for instance, reported that 65% did not have any type of gerontological training at all and more than 80% felt inadequate to work with older persons (Moberg, 1983). A study of Lutheran parishes in the state of New York reported that when the elderly constitute a high percentage of the congregation the pastor may show an interest in, but not an aptitude for, developing a specialized ministry for the elderly (Doka, 1985–1986).

Despite these educational barriers there is great potential for mobilizing the energy of congregational members toward the problems of frailty in old age and toward the caregivers as well. Tobin and colleagues (1986) have identified four broad roles for churches and synagogues: (1) offering religious programs, (2) serving as host, (3) providing pastoral care programs, and (4) offering service programs. Religious institutions already excel at performing some of these services that affect the elderly, such as visiting the shut-in, pastoral counseling, and hosting mutual help groups (which serve a considerable number of persons during midlife or later). In this latter regard, a survey of 2,500 self-help groups revealed that 44% of them met in churches or synagogues, more than in any other community site (Madara & Peterson, 1986). Additional church-based activities could be stimulated by incorporating gerontological education into seminary training (Payne, 1986). Another strategy to stimulate gerontological programs is through community training projects that target congregations and their desire to serve the elderly.

The most widely recognized program for training congregation members to work with the elderly in need is the Shepherd's Center, which began in 1972 in Kansas City, Missouri. Under the auspices of the Central United Methodist Church, the focus of the program has served as a model for similar centers throughout the United States and Canada. Volunteers participate in a training program and choose the type of voluntary activity that will help keep older persons independent. Since the cessation of funds from a 3-year grant from the Missouri State Office on Aging, Shepherd's Center programs are supported by participating churches and synagogues, foundations, and corporations, as well as individual fees and donations.

Another project that has the potential to spawn independent programs around the nation is the Interfaith Volunteer Caregivers Program, cosponsored by the Robert Wood Johnson Foundation, the nation's largest medical care foundation, and the National Interfaith Coalition on Aging. This project has demonstrated around the country that when religious leaders are given the opportunity to host a gerontological program they seize it (Haber, 1988a). The basic objective of the 3-year program was to fund religious coalitions willing to develop innovative programs to serve the frail, isolated elderly in the community. The primary mechanism to serve the elderly was to recruit, train, place, and supervise volunteer caregivers from religious institutions as well as from the larger community.

Over 900 organizational representatives responded to the nationwide announcement. In March 1984, after a year-long selection process, 25 grantees were selected on the basis of their innovative program designs, strong local coalitions, and geographical representation throughout the United States. A major goal of the program was that when it ended, in March 1987, volunteer caregivers would be sustained even though grant monies would be terminated. Project staff were encouraged to form advisory boards to sustain the efforts of volunteer caregivers and to seek alternative modes of funding from the United Way, local foundations, and other sources of public and private support.

Results from the first 2 years of this 3-year project indicated that the 25 grantees organized 10,000 volunteers to serve the needs of 26,000 care recipients (IVCP in perspective, 1986). Eight hundred seventy-five congregations (66% Protestant, 20% Roman Catholic, 1% Jewish, and 13% other) affiliated with these 25 projects. For the most part, volunteers provided transportation, shopping, friendly visiting, advice and referral, telephone reassurance, respite, and meal preparation. To a much lesser extent, more personal and intensive services, such as toileting, feeding, bathing, hospice care, and fiscal management assistance, were provided.

The Washington, D.C., program, which was one of the 25 grantees of the nationwide project, involved a collaboration among four organizations:

1. The Interfaith Conference of Metropolitan Washington is a coalition of four major faith communities—Protestant, Roman Catholic, Jewish, and Islamic—that disseminates information to 1,500 congregations.
2. So Others May Eat is an ecumenical organization to minister to the homeless and other poor through medical, dental, and social services.
3. The Institute of Gerontology at the University of the District of Columbia implements caregiver training programs to frail, noninstitutionalized elderly.
4. The Southeast Vicariate Cluster is a cluster of 15 congregations (mostly Roman Catholic) that provides service and advocacy for the poor minority residents in the southeast quadrant of the District of Columbia.

In brief, the congregation-based caregiving training program in Washington, D.C., consisted of 12 hours of lecture and discussion on such topics as psychological aspects of aging, sensory deprivation, communicating with older persons, choosing among housing alternatives, chronic illness, and accessing community resources (Silverman et al., 1981—see Appendix B for other caregiving manuals). Each participating congregation received a community resource directory. During the last few hours of the training session, trainees were encouraged to form a self-help group to continue to generate educational forums and to access—or generate—caregiving resources both from within the congregation and from the community at large.

By the end of the second year of the project, 317 trainees from 30 Protestant and Catholic congregations completed the 12-hour caregiving training program. Six of the 30 congregations formed ongoing mutual self-help groups. Group members learned how to gain access to expert speakers from the community to address such common problem areas as making a will, managing hypertension, and preventing crime. Each group had a member trained to use a resource directory and to update its listings. Two groups organized ongoing small group discussions to provide emotional support to existing caregivers. One group organized a program to transport elderly to services and other religious events. Another group implemented a senior recognition day.

Comparing the 20% of the congregations ($n = 6$) with mutual help groups and the 80% ($n = 24$) without such groups did not reveal any systematic differences (Haber, 1984b). Formation of a group could not be predicted on the basis of congregation size, percentage of elderly, income level, denomination, and so on. The six successful groups were started by deaconesses and other church leaders who had both a strong interest in caregiving and the leadership skills to sustain a group. Project staff did not have the resources (nor the mandate from the funding agency) to analyze how such skills and interests could be developed in a higher percentage of the congregations.

In addition to church-based training programs and mutual help groups, the

Washington, D.C., program matched volunteers (both from congregations and the community at large) with isolated elders in the community who needed support. By the end of the second year of the project 80 volunteers were recruited, trained, and supervised. Most of the services that were provided were on the order of companionship and minor chore aid. If an elderly care recipient declined in health, referrals were made to homemaker services, the food stamp program, and other social services.

As expected, the matching program identified more isolated elders with service needs than volunteers who were willing to be trained and placed. In addition, more volunteer help was needed to monitor the changing conditions of caregivers and to provide timely referrals and other services. Nonetheless, the basic project goals for both the training program and the volunteer match program were met. The number of participants projected to be reached was achieved, and participant satisfaction in the programs was high.

A dissemination project funded by the Administration on Aging is attempting to replicate the Washington, D.C., program in 100 congregations in the Washington, D.C., metropolitan area—but in a more cost-effective manner, and over a shorter period of time (Fields, 1987). In brief, this train-the-trainer approach will provide an 18-hour caregiving training program to one or two leaders from each of the participating religious institutions. The congregational leaders who participate in the program will receive caregiving curriculum, instructions on how to teach it, a supplementary bibliography, access to a university's gerontology library and speaker's bureau, and ongoing technical assistance as needed from professional staff.

The 18-hour dissemination program is not an attempt to produce caregiving experts. Instead it starts with experienced teachers and leaders in congregations who are interested in caregiving and provides them with the curriculum, supplementary information, access to resource persons, and ongoing educational seminars that will allow them to disseminate useful caregiving information to congregation members.

Finally, in each of the dissemination classes the participants from different faiths will be encouraged to develop relationships among themselves to facilitate further implementation of caregiving programs. Congregations could, for instance, exchange resource persons or implement interfaith projects in the community.

Based on previous projects (Haber, 1984a,b), it is estimated that about 20% of the caregiving training programs will result in ongoing mutual self-help groups. The support groups are likely to be widely disparate in their focus, including those that are oriented internally (i.e., toward the provision of education, discussion, or emotional support to existing members) and those that are community-based volunteer projects. The latter includes such activities as senior escort programs, respite exchanges, and the development and use of a community resource and service directory.

WORK-SITE ELDER CARE PROGRAMS

Approximately one in four workers in America, the great majority of them women, have another job when they get home—taking care of an aging parent. An emerging employee benefit, elder care, is appearing in the work arena to respond to this need. While elder care is not common among major corporations today (Creedon, 1987), one analyst suggests that it may become "the new pioneering benefit of the 1990's" (Friedman, 1986) when the baby boomers surge into their 40s—a prime time for being concerned about caring for an aging parent. Moreover, corporate decisionmakers are most likely to be in this age group and to be caring for an older relative. Thus, employer sympathy for this problem is likely to be heightened.

Employers can already offer a range of elder care programs or benefits to meet the needs of working caregivers. One response would be to link with the federal government's Dependent Care Benefit Plan so that up to $5,000 in pretax wages can be used for the care of dependents, regardless of age. To apply it to elder care, though, the dependent elder must have a gross taxable annual income of less than $1,900 per year, live in the home of the employee at least 8 hours a day, and be dependent on the employee for daily care and over half of his or her financial support.

Another employer response would be to provide employees with caregiving informational packets (developed by the American Association of Retired Persons or the National Association of Area Agencies on Aging—see the list of elder care resources in Appendix B). Additional employer responses are to train counselors working through employee assistance programs to assist with problems associated with aging, to allow employee caregivers to take advantage of flexible work schedules, and to offer day care programs that provide care for children and elderly parents in the same company-sponsored center.

One of the model elder care programs in the nation was developed by the Travelers Corporation in response to an employee survey. The Travelers Corporation has more than 7,000 employees age 30 or older in their home office in Hartford, Connecticut. Employees were randomly polled in June 1985 so that those with major caregiving responsibilities to relatives or friends age 55 or older could be identified. More than one in four respondents (28%) reported they did have caregiving responsibilities, with 27% of these caring for more than one person. Employee caregivers ranged disproportionately between the ages of 41 and 55, as indicated by the fact that, while 37% of Travelers' home office work force was between these ages, 52% of them had caregiving responsibilities.

For those employees age 40 and over, caregiving responsibilities have persisted for an average of 6.5 years. The majority of the care recipients being served had two or more medical problems. More than half of these recipients suffered a major illness or injury that precipitated this need for care. The types of medical problems that 10% or more of the care receivers were coping with were wide ranging: impaired vision, swollen legs/ankles, impaired hearing, arthritis, depression, hypertension, memory loss/disorientation, heart disorders, insomnia, constipation/diarrhea, dizziness/falls, uncontrollable elimination, diabetes, stroke, respiratory problems, and bone fractures/breaks.

More than half of the caregivers reported they helped run the household of the care recipient by performing such chores as cooking, laundry, cleaning, managing finances, and providing transportation. As is typical of caregivers in general, female employees (63%) were much more likely than males (29%) to report they are the primary care provider.

In response to their employee survey results, Travelers developed a model elder care program that consisted of the following informational and educational programs, insurance coverage, and personnel policies:

1. Employees can buy nursing home insurance for themselves, their spouses, or their parents at group rates. American Express offered this program through Travelers Insurance in 1988 for the first time. The amount of the premium depends on the employee's age at entry, and it does not rise with age.
2. A work-site caregiving information fair was implemented, which involved 20 community agencies to provide information on home health care, adult day care, legal and financial help, coping with stress, and so forth. More than 700 employees and retirees attended the first fair.
3. Ten 1-hour lunchtime seminars were offered on a variety of topics, such as family decisionmaking, coping with mental changes, legal considerations, housing choices, and so on. About 60 persons attended these seminars.
4. Self-help groups for caregivers met weekly to share problems and ideas. Two sets of 15 to 20 persons with especially heavy caregiving responsibilities joined the first two groups, led by employee assistance program counselors.
5. Videotaped informational messages on caregiving were shown at viewing booths in several home office locations, with interactive monitors at some of these sites.
6. A series of caregiving articles featuring interviews with experts in the field are planned for upcoming issues of the company newspapers.
7. Caregiving reference materials will be added to the corporate library.
8. Flexible work time schedules have been instituted to accommodate the individual schedules of caregiving employees.
9. A dependent care allowance program automatically deducts pretax dollars from the caregiving employee's paycheck for deposit into a special account exclusively for dependent care expenses.
10. An allowance of up to 4 weeks per year of unpaid personal leave is available to employees.

WORK–SITE WELLNESS

Work-site wellness programs are proliferating nationwide. Corporate leaders are becoming knowledgeable about recent studies that correlate participation in work-site wellness programs with lower absenteeism and tardiness, fewer medical insurance and disability compensation claims, increased productivity because of higher morale, and lower turnover rates (Kizer, 1987). Since working people spend half their waking hours at work, employers are in a good position not only to reduce their medical costs and increase employee productivity, but to act in the best interest of the American public.

Omaha, Nebraska, has been especially innovative in this regard because it was the site for the first wellness council in the country, the Wellness Council of the Midlands (WELCOM), founded in 1982. WELCOM has served as a model for other councils in cities across America (Tucson, Norristown, Atlanta, Chattanooga, Columbus, Jacksonville, Milwaukee, Minneapolis, Greensboro, and Baton Rouge). In 1987 Wellness Councils of America (WELCOA) was founded in Omaha, for the purpose of developing work-site wellness councils throughout America. By March 1988 WELCOM and WELCOA had stimulated the development of wellness councils in 22 cities across America.

WELCOM serves as a clearinghouse for information and resources on work-site wellness in the Greater Omaha area. WELCOM's 120 member companies send delegates to meetings for the purpose of exchanging ideas and resources and offering support for wellness planning and programming. According to founder William Kizer (1987), the Wellness Council reaches out to 70,000 employees of member organizations, their family members, and others—perhaps one third of all persons living in Omaha.

Why *work-site* wellness? As they say in the realty business, three reasons—location, location, and location. Work-site programs have higher participation rates than community programs. Employees need not negotiate transportation nor the time, hassle, and cost involved with programs in other parts of the community. Also work-site programs are responsive to the schedules of employees. In addition, employers can encourage their employees to take advantage of these mutually beneficial programs by giving periodic reminders and stressing the value of health-promoting behaviors.

Why work-site *wellness* councils? Good health is good for the employees, obviously, but also for the employer. An increasing number of studies document improvements in employee health that directly increase corporate profits (see Fig. 5.1).

Smoking cessation programs, for instance, reduce morbidity and mortality rates. Scholl (1980) estimates that one third of deaths occurring in men age 50 to 60 could have been avoided if all smoking had ceased at age 50. Former smokers halve their absentee rates (Kizer, 1987) and reduce their health claims by $300 per annum (New rules of exercise, 1986). Studies of exsmokers age 65

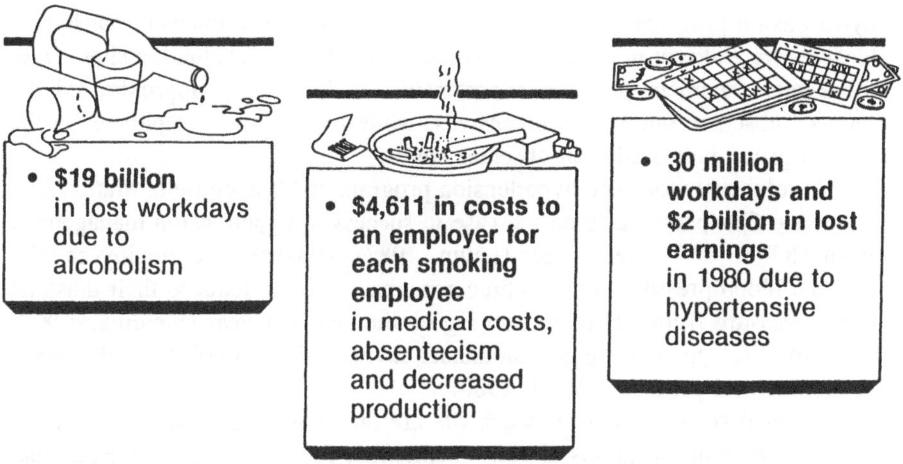

FIGURE 5.1 Costs of unhealthy life-styles. From *Long-term needs of the elderly: A federal-state-private partnership.* (1984). Presented at a hearing before the U.S. Senate Special Committee on Aging, Seattle. Washington, DC: U.S. Government Printing Office.

to 74 indicate that quitting will lower the risk of coronary heart disease to the level of nonsmokers in as few as 1 to 5 years (Jajich, 1984).

Kristen (1980) and Weis (1981) summarize studies that document cost savings from smoking cessation programs ranging between $624 and $4,611 annually per employee in terms of medical costs, absenteeism, replacement costs, maintenance efforts, property damage, other insurance increases, and productivity. A study at Harvard University's School of Public Health reports smoking cessation programs to be the most prevalent wellness program. Many corporations are offering incentives to quit smoking, such as bonuses, rebates, and vacation trips. Creighton University's Health Sciences Center in Omaha, Nebraska, recently joined this growing list of employers offering incentives to foster smoking cessation.

Participants in Control Data Corporation's smoking cessation program in Bloomington, Minnesota, were classified after 1 year as quitters (31%), reducers (at least 50% less—44%) or failures (24%). Those who quit for 5 or more years reduced benefit payments by 25% and halved their number of days as hospital patients compared with those who continued to smoke. Fielding (1982) reviewed smoking cessation programs at the work site and concluded that smoking abstinence rates were at least twice as high as community-based programs.

The National Heart, Lung, and Blood Institute's (1983) demonstration project on *Work Place High Blood Pressure Control* reports that more than 26 million work days are lost each year to cardiovascular disease and hypertension. This institute collaborated with the Ford Motor Company and the University of Michigan's Institute for Labor and Industrial Relations on a work-site hypertension program. Before the program, the study documented that hypertensives were absent more than normotensives at all four evaluation sites. Over the 2-year treatment program hypertensives under control approximated the reduced absentee rate of normotensives, while hypertensive employees in the control group increased their absenteeism.

A voluntary work-site hypertension program at Massachusetts Mutual Life Insurance Company led to an increase in successful hypertension management from 36% to 82% after 1 year (Levin, 1987). Hypertensive employees who attend a blood pressure control clinic near the work site reduced their diastolic blood pressure from 103 to 83 mm Hg by the end of 1 year (Fielding, 1982). New York Telephone estimates an annual savings of $663,000 from its hypertension control program (Wood, 1980).

Medical screenings at the work site are far ranging. In addition to hypertensive screening programs already mentioned, there are tests for glaucoma, colon cancer, obesity, and blood chemistries and other screenings of importance to the aging employee and retiree. IBM instituted a multiphasic screening program targeted to employees 35 years of age and older. The battery of tests is repeated every 5 years or more often if necessary. Interestingly, if not surprisingly, 41% of those screened identified medical conditions for the first time (Beck, 1986).

Exercise programs are impacting positively on the health of older workers as well as retirees. Occidental Life Insurance Company and Northern Natural Gas Company reported reduced absenteeism as a consequence of their fitness programs (Levin, 1987). Hodgson and Buskirk (1977) documented the positive impact of an exercise program on cardiovascular function in the elderly. DeVries (1970) and Sidney et al. (1977) reported that regardless of an elderly person's prior exercise habits, an appropriate aerobic exercise program will increase maximum oxygen consumption between 10% and 30%. Studies of regular exercise programs with the elderly report decreases in systolic and diastolic blood pressure (Buccola & Stone, 1975; deVries, 1970; Haber, 1983, 1986a). Also, elderly subjects placed on a low-intensity exercise program substantially increased their bone mineral content (Krolner et al., 1983; Smith, 1982).

A substantial number of employers are providing exercise and fitness programs. The vast majority of these, however, are high-intensity programs (aerobic dance, weight lifting programs, sports, etc.) most suitable to younger employees. A high-intensity exercise program is beneficial to younger employees but is dangerous for many older employees. A low-intensity exercise program (such as low-impact aerobic dance) may, in fact, be high-intensity to an older person or to a younger person at a less-than-average fitness level for his or her age.

While not aging oriented, some innovative fitness programming has been conducted. Hospital Corporation of America, for instance, pays employees for each "aerobic unit" performed. Citibank provides seminars on warm-up techniques, how to select appropriate running shoes, and how to develop an exercise regimen. Ford offers mileage measurements for employees who choose to take brisk walks indoors during breaks (Levin, 1987).

The importance of calcium balance and calcium requirements on preventing osteoporosis has been studied by Dr. Robert Heaney and colleagues (1977) at Creighton University of Omaha, Nebraska. Other researchers have documented a link between dietary habits and cardiovascular disease as well as a reduction in salt intake with lower blood pressure levels (Izzo, 1982; Puska et al., 1983; Rouse et al., 1983).

Nutritional programs based on research findings are increasingly being offered at the work site. Some companies offer a special healthy menu, while others provide nutritional information, such as caloric and cholesterol content of food in their cafeterias (Kiefhaber & Goldbeck, 1986). Overweight employees at Pioneer Hi-Bred receive five dollars per pound lost until a desired weight is reached. If the new weight is maintained for a year, the employee has a choice of gifts valued at about $75. Half of the overweight employees have lost weight through this program (Kiefhaber & Goldbeck, 1986).

While work-site wellness appears to be of interest to large and small businesses alike, the motivation to initiate a program may vary by the size of the business. Large companies are especially concerned about the health expenditures generated by employees. Chrysler Chairman Lee Iacocca was the first to calculate how much employee health care costs added to the cost of a product. Iacocca reported his astonishment to learn that approximately $600 was added to the price of each car that Chrysler sold (Califano, 1986). Through a combination of cost containment factors, including wellness programs, Chrysler reduced its health care costs by $58 million in 1984 alone. Since U.S. companies nationwide paid out more than $87 billion in health insurance premiums for their employees, retirees, and their dependents in 1985, there is a strong motivation for them to do what is necessary to keep people healthy.

On a small business level, work-site wellness programs are initiated mainly for human resource management reasons (*Healthworks,* 1984). Employee morale, absenteeism, job turnover rate, and other factors that affect productivity can be changed through inexpensive wellness programs. Through a targeted health information program and knowledge of free or low-cost services in the community, small businesses can benefit with a very modest outlay of funds.

Do the programs work? In the Omaha area, Kizer (1987) reports that the Creighton University health program for Omaha Police Department officers lowered coronary risks, Central States of Omaha employees collectively lost 285 pounds, Valmont Industries reduced turnover rates among personnel and reduced medical costs as well, Millard Manufacturing lowered absenteeism among employees, and Metropolitan Utilities District in Omaha reported that over 70% of their female employees attended a seminar on breast cancer conducted by the American Cancer Society.

WORK–SITE WELLNESS AND AGING

In 1987 a national health promotion survey reported that health promotion programs have become so popular that one of every two work sites is engaged in some type of health promotion (Erikson, 1987). While work-site wellness programs are proliferating nationwide, age has not been used as a basis for the establishment of the vast majority of programs. Nonetheless, demographic changes in the work force are making this shift imperative. The Labor Department, for example, reports that employees age 35 to 54 will represent the greatest percentage increase in the work force over the next decade (Fullerton & Tschetter, 1983). As the work force grows older, the median age of employees will rise from age 32 in 1980 to age 42 by the year 2030 (Levin, 1987). Already many long-established businesses have work forces that average in the 40s.

At the same time the work force is aging, retirees are both expanding in number and growing older. Among major employers the ratio of three active employees for each retiree is fast becoming the norm (Levin, 1987). This contrasts markedly with American corporations as recently as 1960, when the ratio was at least 10 to 1. In the industrial sector, employee layoffs have increased while average retirement age and new hiring rates have been lowered. The support ratio of workers to retirees in these industries is about 1 to 1 (Levin, 1987). The significance of a growing retiree population is based in large part on the escalating unfunded liability for retiree health care. Currently estimated at between $125 billion to $2 trillion, this liability will grow rapidly as the population ages and as the federal government attempts to transfer costs to employers (Polich et al., 1987).

As the nation and employees age, the prevalence of chronic conditions increases. Comparing younger workers (under age 45), for example, with older workers (age 45 to 64) and retirees, the following trends emerge: Arthritis is 5 times more likely among older workers and 10 times more likely among retirees, hypertension 5 times more likely among older workers and 7 times among retirees, hearing impairments 5 times more likely among older workers and 7 times among retirees, heart conditions 3 times more likely among older workers and 7 times among retirees, and diabetes 6 times more likely among older workers and 10 times among retirees (Newquist, 1985). What makes the presence of these chronic conditions significant is the association of these conditions with increased number of physician visits, more frequent and longer hospital stays, and increased use of medications (National Center for Health Statistics, 1986).

Despite this epidemiological mandate, work-site wellness programs may discriminate against older workers and retirees in favor of programming to younger adults. Younger workers going out for the company sports team may intimidate the older worker. Popular aerobic dance classes may not be "low impact" enough to suit the tastes of older workers, and the music may not be appealing. A survey of employee benefit specialists documented the existence of age discrimination—three out of four specialists asserted that their wellness programs appealed primarily to those who need them the least—the younger and healthier workers (International Society of Certified Employe Benefit Specialists, 1985).

Another reason work-site wellness programs may be skewed toward the younger employee is that most health promotion staff are young themselves. "At General Electric, Campbell Soup and Johnson and Johnson, the average age of staff members is less than 30. This is typical for fitness center staff; it is rare to find instructors over the age of 40" (Levin, 1987). It is questionable whether youth-oriented program staff members understand the special needs and interests of older employees or retirees. Levin (1987) notes that there are reports of older employees and retirees resenting the condescending attitudes of younger health promotion staff toward them.

Yet another reason for the exclusion of older persons is limited resources. Only 15% of companies with wellness programs permit retirees to participate (Business and health, 1985). Possible reasons are space limitations, added staff costs, possible legal liability, and mere lack of consideration (i.e., no one thinks to extend an invitation).

Preretirement programs may be a promising direction for work-site wellness initiatives. Survey information indicates that these planning programs are on the rise, from the two thirds of major employers who are currently offering preretirement programs (Business and health, 1985) to the projected three quarters by 1989 (Segal, 1986). Moreover, these programs continue to lower the eligibility age, which has traditionally been set at 55. More companies are adopting "life planning" or career planning to begin in the 40s or even earlier. In addition, a few of these preretirement programs are adding a wellness component to their content (Levin, 1987). The adoption of wellness has moved the preretirement programs out of the exclusive domain of the personnel director and into the company medical and health department program.

For the most part, age-responsive programming targets persons age 40 and over. From the corporate perspective, age 40 has been designated as the minimum age for legal protection against age discrimination in the areas of hiring, promotion, and dismissal (the federal government's Age Discrimination in Employment Act). From the perspective of prevention and health promotion, age 40 begins the decade when changes in sensory capacity are noticeable (hearing and vision especially), and the reserve capacity of the major physical systems is less responsive to stressors (Saxon & Etten, 1987). From the perspective of the caregiver, the decade of the 40s is the beginning of a major caregiving role for an adult child with an aging parent.

Age-responsive programming can extend down into the decades of the 20s and 30s, also. Some of these employees, for example, are confronting the caregiving issue with grandparents or parents. In addition, these younger persons may not be in good physical shape. Thus, a low-impact aerobics class may be just as appropriate for a younger worker needing rehabilitation as an older employee or retiree seeking more gentle physical activity.

Also, some younger employees may have a family history of hypertension, cancer, diabetes, heart disease, or stroke. While medical screenings in these areas are typically recommended on an annual or biannual basis for older persons, they may be quite helpful for younger persons with familial disease in these areas or who are prematurely contending with a chronic health condition.

SURVEYING CORPORATE WELLNESS PROGRAMS

On a national level the Washington Business Group on Health (WBGH), the first national employer association dedicated to medical care cost management, represents more than 200 of the nation's largest employers. These employers are responsible for providing health care to more than 50 million employees, retirees, and dependents. As part of its information services the WBGH has compiled a list of 26 large employer health programs for older workers and retirees. A few examples of corporate health promotion programs with an aging emphasis are noted below (Creedon, 1987; Levin, 1987):

Levi Straus & Company

- Provides medical screening that includes diabetes and colorectal cancer screening and blood pressure measurements.
- Newsletter *Arucuate* provides health information on nutrition, exercise, stress management, and so forth.

Tenneco

- Developed four 1-hour courses for its older workers on subjects such as arthritis, osteoporosis, and nutrition.
- Developed a course called Aerobic Light, for midlife women.
- Offers a sport activity called Wallyball, a modified version of volleyball especially popular with older workers.
- Forty percent of employees age 40 and over participate in fitness center activities.

System Development Corporation

- Provides medical screening for carotid duples scanning for plaque buildup on the carotid artery.
- Developed a nutrition program given each month that includes a home-cooked meal and instructions on how to prepare the food.

Kimberly-Clark Corporation

- Developed seminars called Women and Mid-Life Health.

Offers water exercise classes called Aquacize that appeal to older adults and retirees with arthritis or back problems.

The Travelers Company

Offers a retiree employment program that places retirees in part-time and temporary jobs in the company.

Provides employee caregiving programs offering educational seminars on caregiving, support groups, and flexible work hours.

Pitney Bowes, Inc.

Offers a support group for caregivers at the work site, and trains employee assistance counselors regarding elder care issues.

Pepsico, Inc.

Developed a manual for employees called *Eldercare.*

Conducted programs and set up a "hot-line" program, linked to a local center on aging, for the employee-caregiver.

Pfizer

Recruited more than half of its women employees age 55 and over to participate in a special screening and fitness programs at its corporate headquarters in New York.

While these programs are too new and few in number to produce any firm conclusions, there are several common elements that appear to contribute to successful corporate programs (Haber & Wicht, 1987; Levin, 1987):

1. A substantive focus on common chronic illnesses, such as osteoporosis, arthritis, diabetes, hypertension, and so on, may attract more employees in an aging work force.
2. Knowledgeable and enthusiastic staff who are trained for working with older adults and have good communication skills may be more responsive to an aging work force.
3. Spouse eligibility can build enthusiasm, especially with certain behavior modification programs such as smoking cessation and nutrition.
4. Overall health risk appraisals may uncover conditions or behaviors that place an employee at risk.
5. Recognition of individual achievement and highlighting personal fitness goals may increase motivational levels.
6. Preretirement planning programs are popular and can provide a relatively uncontroversial framework in which age can be used as a criterion for program recruitment and development.
7. Appealing to mid-life workers in their 40s and 50s may be more effective through responsive programming, rather than rigid age requirements that may be viewed as stigmatizing.

6

PROFESSIONAL CAREGIVERS

Health professionals are formal caregivers; that is, they have completed a systematic and rigorous series of courses in their chosen field. Most professionals today, however, whether they are practitioners in the community or faculty in the university, have never been formally trained in geriatrics. In fact, most professionals have not had a single course on how to provide the care required by older persons. The National Institute on Aging (1987) reports that while attention to geriatrics in the educational programs of most health professions has expanded in recent years, the "current number of prepared teaching faculty and investigators ranges from only 5 to 25 percent (depending on the field) of the total number estimated to be needed for the development of such activities."

NEED FOR DISCIPLINARY GERIATRIC EDUCATION WITHIN DISCIPLINES

The need for geriatric medical education was succinctly summarized by Bennett and colleagues (1986). In 1984 clinical programs in geriatrics "did not exist in 35 percent of departments of internal medicine, 41 percent of departments of family practice and 50 percent of departments of psychiatry. Only slightly more than two percent of third- and fourth-year medical students enrolled in geriatrics courses." Moreover, what little geriatric content does reach the medical student is highly specialized, and makes no reference to the complex, interrelated problems that characterize the elderly patient.

A 1981 survey of dental schools found that more than half of all schools did not have any geriatric content in their dental school curricula. Only seven schools had formal courses (Ettinger et al., 1981; Thomas & Ship, 1981).

A 1982 survey by the National Association of Social Workers revealed that only 5% of the 50,000 trained social workers indicated that service to the elderly was their primary interest with another 1% reporting it to be a secondary interest (National Institute on Aging, 1984).

Nurses have substantial responsibilities providing services to the elderly in hospitals, nursing homes, and in the community. Not surprisingly, almost all nursing education programs include content related to the elderly (Knowles, 1982). The major obstacle to geriatric nursing education, however, is the inadequate preparation of faculty. Most of the existing nursing faculty have been self-taught or limited to a few continuing education courses (National Institute on Aging, 1984).

Of 72 pharmacy schools surveyed, 22% had no geriatric content, 35% offered minimal geriatric content, and 43% offered at least one course with geriatrics as a primary focus (Simonson & Pratt, 1982). Among those courses offered, many were without a clinical component or were offered as electives that most students did not take because of concentrated class schedules. Thus, the majority of pharmacy students are graduating with inadequate preparation for a population that consumes more than 25% of the prescriptions dispensed (Simonson & Pratt, 1982).

Older persons are seen as a special population for counseling, and the need for counseling strategies with older adults has been acknowledged (Myers & Blake, 1986). A study conducted in 1981, however, reports that two thirds of counselor education departments nationwide do not offer coursework to train counselors to work with older people (Myers, 1983). While much work has been done to train counselors in gerontology since 1975, when only 6% of all counselor education programs even offered an elective in aging, the vast majority of counselors today have received no geriatric preparation.

INTERDISCIPLINARY GERIATRIC EDUCATION

The authors of two landmark works, *The Structure of Scientific Revolutions* (Kuhn, 1970) and *Double Helix* (Watson, 1968), document the importance of interdisciplinary collaboration behind many of the breakthroughs in the history of science. An interdisciplinary approach to research or education occurs when disciplinary professionals meet to work jointly on areas of overlapping concern. Responsibilities are assigned on the basis of individual competence and access to information rather than traditional disciplinary affiliations.

In contrast, a multidisciplinary approach is similar to the parallel play of children—while everyone may work (or play) together, there is limited awareness of what the others are doing. Each disciplinary professional is, in fact, careful not to trespass on the territories of others. Regarding geriatric education, the physician Herman Blumenthal noted in a 1965 issue of *The Gerontologist* that after 20 years of effort through a gerontological society there was a proliferation of multidisciplinary conferences, journals, and symposia, but scientists still wound up communicating exclusively with colleagues in their own disciplines.

Twenty years later, there is a resurgence of interest in interdisciplinary activity. The multiple, intertwined, and chronic health problems of older persons make the teaching of teamwork skills critically important in the preparation of health care professionals (National Institute on Aging, 1984). To meet this challenge Interdisciplinary Team Training in Geriatrics (ITTG) programs have been set up in Veterans Administration hospitals around the country. The director of the program, Jan Frezell, reports that it is too early to tell what kind of impact the ITTG program is having on the staff or patients in the VA system (personal communication, 1986).

In the educational arena, the Association of Gerontology in Higher Education has recently convened a committee on interdisciplinary education. Dr. David Satin, the committee's chair and a physician at Harvard's Medical School, reports that "Interdisciplinary education is often lauded, sometimes required, but seldom accomplished in practice" (1986).

A review of the literature reveals a consensus on the barriers affecting the development of interdisciplinary collaboration:

1. Disciplinary territoriality (Spence et al., 1986)
2. Different knowledge bases and beliefs on how knowledge is to be accumulated and understood (Shriner et al., 1983)
3. Difficulty understanding or supporting the goals of interdisciplinary education by college deans and department chairpersons (Satin, 1986)
4. Disagreement over when interdisciplinary education should be introduced into the student's curriculum (Nichols, 1981)
5. Conflict regarding equal status among disciplines (Satin, 1986)
6. Disagreement on how (or whether) faculty should be rewarded in the development or implementation of programs (Treants et al., 1981)
7. Disagreement on how teamwork skills should be introduced into the clinical training of students (Spence et al., 1986)
8. Conflict in the coordination of learning experiences among the different disciplines (Molinari et al., 1983)

On an individual level, as people grow older their needs become more complex and interdependent. Failing physical health, for instance, will limit the mobility of older persons and their capacity to maintain a social support network. Similarly, inadequate finances (and insurance) will limit the capacity of an older person to access long-term care services in order to maintain independence at home. A breakdown in one system, therefore, whether it is physical, economical, social, psychological, or cognitive, is likely to affect the others.

The same interdependency holds true within any one system. Focusing on physical health, for instance, a younger person's broken bone must be set. The older person's hip fracture, however, may require a surgeon, an examination for osteoporosis, an "activity of daily living" assessment by both a therapist and a social worker, and the likely intervention of other health care professionals. Within the health arena alone, there are more than 200 different types of health personnel providing services to the elderly (Shepard et al., 1985). The competent professional must know when to refer a patient to another professional, to whom the patient should be referred, and also how to collaborate in areas of shared knowledge and skills.

From the perspective of administrators at institutes of higher education, the interdisciplinary challenge is substantial as well. We have entered the era of burgeoning specializations, rigid professional boundaries, and the hoarding of resources due to a weakened economy (Scott et al., 1983). Much of the power of the health sciences, moreover, comes from a reductionist model that separates medical components. It follows, therefore, that the university's administrative structure compartmentalizes its curricula, students, faculty, and administrators (Cole, 1983; Gadow, 1983).

Even within disciplines there is a tendency to compartmentalize subject matter. For instance, while educational programs in geriatric care and disease prevention are on the rise, there has been inadequate integration between the two areas. A 1983 survey of medical schools by Simson and Wilson, for instance, found that there were 143 courses that had content on aging and 484 courses with a disease prevention component. Only 20 courses, however, had aging *and* disease prevention. Geriatric disease prevention is not integrated in the curriculum despite the fact that physicians spend 25% of patient care time on education and counseling. Simson and Wilson's (1983) survey of 4-year BA programs in nursing revealed similar findings. While 39 courses had aging content and 190 courses had disease prevention content, only 25 had both aging and disease prevention material.

Finally, while the hospital, the traditional clinical site for health student training, constitutes a multidisciplinary setting, interdisciplinary team training is almost nonexistent (Blumenfield et al., 1982). There is a reluctance to experiment with innovative health care approaches in the hospital setting and an overreliance on the hospital site for student training (Scott et al., 1983). Clinical training activities in hospitals and other acute care clinical settings invariably involve the medical model, with a focus on disease, cure, and physician-dominated team meetings (Spence et al., 1986).

GERIATRIC EDUCATION CENTERS

With the addition of nine new centers in 1987, there are 31 regional centers of geriatric education funded by the U.S. Public Health Service, Bureau of Health Professions. The purpose of the centers is to train health professions' faculty and practitioners in geriatric health care, with an emphasis on the multidisciplinary nature of geriatric practice.

Each geriatric education center (GEC) is charged with the responsibility of training professionals in a range of disciplines, including some of the following frequently served disciplines: medicine, dentistry, pharmacy, nursing, counseling, social work, physical therapy, occupational therapy, nutrition, public health, health education or administration, pastoral counseling, speech and communication, optometry, podiatry, special education, and public administration.

The two major thrusts of the geriatric center are training programs and resource centers. The training programs vary from in-depth educational experiences to short workshops. An example of the former is the 1-year, 60-hour faculty development program at one of the GECs in Pennsylvania. Also, GECs sponsor intensive didactic and clinical training programs through 1-week to 2-month long summer institutes. The more in-depth educational experiences attempt to produce a ripple effect whereby graduates are encouraged to reproduce the educational experience with colleagues and students at their own academic institutes or service agencies.

The other strategy is to offer brief, convenient educational forums (workshops, lectures, conferences, videotapes, teleconferences) in order to reach busy faculty and practitioners who have short blocks of time available in which to target narrow objectives. The focus of these educational forums is on accessibility, specific learning objectives, and limited technical assistance follow-up.

The resource centers associated with the GECs are diverse in purpose and scope. Some publish their own resource catalogues (audiovisual, instructional materials, expert providers, speaker's bureau, journals, etc.). Others develop and disseminate instructional packages to design or integrate gerontological content into new or existing curricula. Most compile or access annotated bibliographies, publish quarterly or semiannual newsletters, offer information and referral services, and conduct computerized bibliographic searches (including the increasingly popular—but expensive—data base AgeLine, which is available through the American Association of Retired Persons).

The original goal of the Bureau of Health Professions, which was started in the 1960s, was to increase the supply of health practitioners in the United States. After World War II the population was growing more quickly than the supply of trained health professionals. In the 1980s and into the future, however, the focus has shifted and will shift from more health professionals to more responsive health professionals. Given the changing demographic reality, health professionals must be better trained in geriatric care.

Better training in geriatrics is more than just content and practical skills. It requires interdisciplinary communication. The major problems that impact on the elderly crosscut disciplinary boundaries. Persons afflicted with arthritis, Alzheimer's disease, and the many health problems associated with age cannot be treated within a specific discipline. There are approximately 30 separate professions of crucial significance to the geriatric patient (Besdine, 1987) and, thus, to the geriatric practitioner. Moreover, many health settings, such as the hospital, nursing home, ambulatory care center, psychiatric facility, and rehabilitation unit, are organized in whole or in part through interdisciplinary teams. Only in the university setting do the strict disciplinary boundaries tend to rule supreme.

A communication challenge, however, exists in the community as well. While many agencies have internal interdisciplinary components, they may not coordinate well with other related agencies in the health, social service, or aging sectors, nor with institutes of higher education. Thus, the GECs can play a catalytic role in this regard. The first step is to define the needs of a local constituency and then develop an action plan for cooperating agencies and organizations to meet those needs. Trust and communication among agencies and organizations can be improved through jointly sponsored conferences, the development of a speaker's bureau, and collaboration on such projects as a geriatric resource bank or continuing education workshops.

CREIGHTON CENTER FOR HEALTHY AGING

It is no longer unusual to see a physician's or dentist's office in a shopping mall. Moreover, it is quite common to see a pharmacy in a shopping mall. Thus, at first glance, the Creighton Center for Healthy Aging (CCHA) located in Omaha, Nebraska, is a not-too-unique combination of health services, with a pharmacy fronting public mall space and a medical and dental complex of offices behind it.

What is unique about the CCHA is its emphasis on health rather than disease. The educational seminar room seats about 40 to 45, and program content is typically on the topics of health promotion, disease prevention, self-care, or maintaining independence. The staff pharmacist, physician, dentist, geriatric nurse practitioner, geriatric social worker, and counselor are frequently among the presenters in the seminar room, though outside expertise is often called on. The educational emphasis extends into the pharmacy, with free printouts of a medication's interaction effects, side effects, compliance suggestions, and the like.

Educational programs are often interdisciplinary in nature. Programs are targeted either to laypersons—typically midlifers or older persons—or to a professional audience. The CCHA houses a geriatric education center—the

Creighton Regional Geriatric Education Center—which services seven health disciplines (and related professions) in Nebraska and eastern Wyoming.

CCHA's research, demonstration, and service projects also focus on health promotion and independence. The Worksite Wellness project (funded by the Health Future Foundation), for instance, focuses on midlife employees (age 40 and over) and retirees seeking caregiving assistance or age-relevant health promotion (such as low-impact aerobic dance classes or nutrition after 50 programs). The Self Care Center (also funded by the Health Future Foundation) provides 7-week series of self-care classes that emphasize living independently with specific chronic diseases (arthritis, hypertension, etc.). Finally, the interdisciplinary geriatric assessment program focuses on maintaining or enhancing functioning in the home setting. In addition to medical assessments, the program includes family consultation, individual counseling, case management, and computerized record-keeping to monitor chronic health conditions.

Since the CCHA is affiliated with a teaching hospital and a university's school of health sciences, training is provided to students in a broad array of disciplines: pharmacy, medicine, dentistry, nursing, allied health, social work, and counseling. The goal of the training program is to involve these students with interdisciplinary teams delivering health services or educational programs. In addition, students are encouraged to include geriatric health promotion as part of their training experience.

The CCHA attempts to apply its health focus as broadly as possible. In addition to affiliating with a wide variety of traditional academic health disciplines, the center reaches out to congregations to provide an annual conference on spiritual well-being and aging; to the work setting with the work-site wellness research and demonstration project; to the family with adult children and spousal caregiver courses; and to state legislators and other politicians through conferences, advocacy efforts, and educational classes.

While the center has no direct competition with other organizations in its broad mission, it does compete with hospitals, universities, outpatient clinics, assessment centers, individual practitioners, health agencies, social service agencies, and other community organizations in the delivery of educational programs and health services, as well as in the acquisition of grants. For this reason, and the fact that it is university affiliated, the accent of the CCHA is on innovation and responding to new societal demands, demographical realities, and economic mandates. Innovative activities, however, can require greater educational responsibilities, as the center attempts to shape consumer demand as well as respond to it.

Another challenge for CCHA is subsidizing educational programs for health promotion and promoting independence for people with chronic conditions. These activities are not reimbursed through traditional insurance programs (though they are part of some health maintenance organizations' package of services), and consumers can find many of these educational programs offered for free in the community. Many hospitals, for example, treat educational programs as a loss leader in order to widen their base of familiarity with area residents, as well as contact with health professionals. Ironically, promoting health, reducing medication usage, and strengthening independence can lead to lower use of hospitals, physicians, dentists, and pharmacies. Thus, health professionals involved with health promotion are engaging in activities designed to reduce business.

Locating a health center in a shopping mall does offer a distinct advantage for marketing programs and services. The Center Shopping Mall, in which the CCHA is located, offers ample free covered parking. Maximum accessibility is also achieved through its bus hub location and geographical centrality (in Omaha) to midlife and older persons. In the eight zip code areas surrounding the CCHA, the heaviest concentration of older persons (23,000 persons age 51 and over) reside in Omaha. The average shopper in the mall in which the CCHA is located is 10 years older than customers of any other shopping mall in the metropolitan area.

Another distinct feature of the CCHA is its consumer-driven emphasis. Through feedback on educational programs, questionnaires to mall customers and community groups, and advice from a community advisory group, the center seeks to be responsive to the community in which it is located. Also, each staff person is encouraged to make community presentations in neighborhood senior centers, service organizations, religious institutions, and schools.

The educational mission of the center, has a multipronged approach. First, the center offers a wide variety of one-time workshops and series of classes for the layperson. At the present time the center is seeking a sponsor for this program, preferably a nearby hospital or a department store that is a neighbor in the mall. Since the center is long on expertise and short on capital, a joint educational effort seems appropriate.

Recently, educational programs for older persons in department stores and other locations in shopping malls have been implemented and found to be enormously successful. While there are many educational programs conducted at senior citizen centers, university campuses, hospitals, and other traditional institutional settings, they, to be blunt, are not attractive to many older persons. Senior centers and nutritional sites can have the stigma of a social welfare program. Universities can be uncomfortably age segregated. And hospitals lack the comfort and enjoyment that a shopping center provides.

The OASIS (Older Adults Service and Information System) program is an example of a shopping mall-based educational program that has been established in 10 department stores owned by the May Company. The flagship program that started in St. Louis, Missouri, in 1982 now has 17,000 members participating in a variety of recreational, educational, social, and cultural activities. Recently, openings of these programs around the country have met with great enthusiasm, including programs in Akron, Ohio; Portland, Oregon;

Washington, D.C.; Cleveland, Ohio; Denver, Colorado; Baltimore, Maryland; and Los Angeles, California. The average age of OASIS program participants is 70, with the range from 60 to 98.

These shopping mall-based educational and information ventures involve collaborative efforts between the May Company store in each of these cities and medical schools, aging agencies, service organizations, or social service agencies.

> *The May Company stores have a commitment to community involvement and a belief that a major department store, as an established institution in the community, has a social responsibility to that community and an image to maintain. It assumes an obligation to the many people who have been loyal customers for many years. The company also is well aware that the percentage of the population over 60 years of age is growing rapidly, and that older adults are more mobile, more financially independent, and better educated. The support of OASIS by the department store is, we believe, an outstanding example of enlightened business thinking. (Older Adults Service and Information System, 1986)*

To serve the needs of midlife and older persons in Omaha a similar joint venture is being pursued.

Second, there is a focus on congregations and corporations. Work and religion are two of our primary institutions, and work-site wellness and spiritual well-being programs, as previously described, are both held at the CCHA and in the community.

Third, as a teaching institution we focus on student training. An internship or clinical rotation at the center provides the student with a unique health emphasis, not to mention an interdisciplinary team approach.

Fourth, we sponsor and organize conferences, holding them both in the shopping mall (seating up to 120 people) and at other sites. The vast majority of mall-based conference participants enjoy the setting and are not distracted by the coming and going of consumers. For conferences in the community we place strong emphasis on collaborating with other agencies, such as the American Association of Retired Persons, the county health department, and the state and area agencies on aging.

Fifth, through the Creighton Regional Geriatric Education Center we provide faculty and professional educational and training programs. Our target groups are physicians, nurses, pharmacists, dentists, occupational therapists, counselors, and social workers in Nebraska and eastern Wyoming.

In short, what sets the CCHA apart from other health services is its multifaceted support of midlife and older persons through interdisciplinary educational, service, and research programs that affect independence and health, not just the treatment of disease.

III

COST-CONSCIOUS SELF-CARE APPROACHES

7

HEALTH PROMOTION AND AGING

In an era of health care cost containment, the most effective way to marshal limited resources is to keep people as healthy as possible. Healthy people use hospitals and nursing homes less, require less professional care and informal caregiving, and, money aside, enjoy life more. The premises on which this section is based are that health promotion is a multifaceted concept that includes—but goes way beyond the boundaries of—the field of medicine and that health promotion is most appropriate for older persons.

During the first half of the 20th century there have been dramatic discoveries that benefited public health, (e.g., immunization, sterilization procedures to improve surgery, antibiotics, and other modes of combating acute disease). As we approach the end of the 20th century, however, American medicine must once again undergo a transformation to benefit the public good. The medical model of care has been based on two premises: that disease is viewed as a deviation from the biomedical norm and that society has the resources to return people to the health status that existed prior to disease or injury.

Older people, on the other hand, will not have all of their diseases cured. Most of their diseases are chronic and must be coped with, without hope of cure. About 90% of the age 65 and over segment of the population, in fact, have at least one chronic condition, and many have multiple noncurable diseases. Moreover, in an aging society, there are not enough public resources to meet all the needs associated with these diseases. Chronic diseases require family and community supports to maintain independence; health promotion and prevention to delay the onset and severity of disease; and also adequate

Social Security, Medicare, and Medicaid benefits to provide alternatives to institutional care. In the upcoming decades biological and biomedical solutions cannot take precedence over the social, economic, and health policy changes that are needed to be responsive to an aging society.

Since shortly before the first surgeon general's report (1979) on the harmful consequences of certain life-styles, we have witnessed a decade of effective behavioral and social change. Cigarette smoking has been significantly curtailed nationwide, with millions having stopped smoking during the past 2 decades; alcohol abuse has been more extensively identified, alcohol support group strategies have been strengthened, and concerned citizens are waging a war against drunk drivers; jogging, aerobic dancing, and other exercises have attracted 20 to 30 million new participants, with the percentage of adults who exercise regularly increasing 100% between the 1960s and the 1980s; better diets are being adopted by a growing number of Americans, with consumption of saturated fats having been reduced markedly, and body weight at a given height having been lowered; seat belt use has been rising steadily, with an increasing percentage of states having adopted seat belt legislation; an increasing number of assertiveness training courses have been combating pathological passivity; and hypertension has been extensively identified and treated in a variety of effective ways, so that heart disease has been reduced by 36% and the incidence of stroke by 40% (Turner, 1985; Weiler, 1983).

The impact of behavioral and social change on health over the past 2 decades has been measurable, with life expectancy for the 65 and over age group increasing 11.6% (Weiler, 1983).

> *Although there is little hope for cure of chronic diseases through the traditional medical model, the onset of these diseases may be postponed through modification of risk factors, many of which are possible to control, either personally or socially. As the onset is delayed to older ages and approaches the limit of the human life span, we can envision a society where everyone can expect to live in vigorous health to close to the average life span and then die after a brief period of illness. (Fries & Crapo, 1986)*

Generally speaking, Americans have taken the 1979 surgeon general's report, *Healthy People,* to heart—literally, since heart disease is the number one killer. The report claims that as much as half of the country's mortality and ill health is due to behavior that could be under individual control, while less than 10% is due to access to medical care. Nonetheless, 97% of all money earmarked by the government for health care in America has been spent for medical treatment (see Fig. 7.1). Modifying life-styles, such as changing exercise habits and diet, has been primarily left to individual initiative.

Health promotion and prevention refer to a wide variety of activities, including exercise, nutrition, stress management, medical self-care, accident pre-

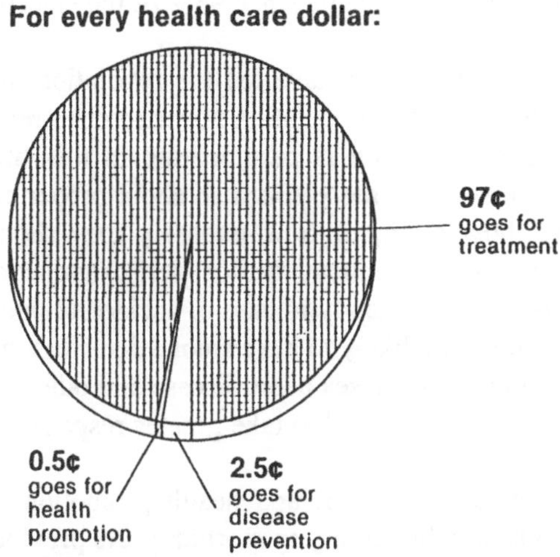

FIGURE 7.1 Health promotion: An ignored priority. From *Long-term needs of the elderly: A federal-state-private partnership.* (1984). Presented at a hearing before the U.S. Senate Special Committee on Aging, Seattle. Washington, DC: U.S. Government Printing Office.

vention, health appraisals, and medical screenings. A national survey conducted in 1982 (Dychtwald, 1986) reported that more than half of all senior centers are sponsoring some type of health promotion or illness-prevention activity. Older persons were going to these centers for exercise programs; nutrition classes; screenings for hypertension, diabetes, glaucoma, and gynecological disorders; mental health counseling; physical health counseling; health education lectures and handouts; physical examinations; and so forth. In short, many senior centers and other community sites where older persons congregate around the nation are turning into wellness centers.

Recent studies have begun to document the areas in which the elderly and the young have asserted leadership in the areas of health promotion and disease prevention (Bausell, 1986; Thornberry et al., 1986). In some areas the elderly have led the way; in other areas they lag behind their younger counterparts. The elderly are in the lead, for example, when it comes to eating sensibly. They are more likely to restrict salt, fat, cholesterol, and sugar; they are more likely to consume fiber, vitamins, minerals, and calcium. In addition, the elderly are more consistent about eating breakfast than other age groups. They are more likely to discuss their eating habits with health care professionals. The elderly drink less alcohol and smoke less tobacco (perhaps because nonsmokers and nondrinkers are more likely to survive to old age). Finally, cases of untreated hypertension have decreased 10% between 1962 and 1974 (Weiler, 1983), and the older person is largely responsible since 93% of the elderly now check their blood pressure regularly.

On the other hand, the young have led the revolution in exercising regularly. While almost half the adult population now exercises regularly, only about a quarter of the older population is participating in this fitness renaissance. Moreover, younger persons are more educated about proper exercising, that is, knowing how long, how often, or how intensely they should exercise. The young are more knowledgeable about medical self-examinations and are more likely to have a phone number handy in case of accidental poisoning. They also use seat belts more, are more likely to have smoke detectors in their homes, and are more likely to know what causes heart disease and other medical problems.

The elderly must be encouraged to take greater responsibility for their own health for two reasons:

1. Self-care, illness prevention, and health promotion are activities that influence an individual's vulnerability to morbidity. As previously summarized, the wellness revolution appears to be impacting positively in this regard on the health of Americans of all ages. However, the elderly take the lead in some health areas and need encouragement in others.

2. Increased responsibility for one's own health is a form of empowerment for the elderly (Spence et al., 1986) that leads to more choices and more satisfaction. This, in turn, can lead to improved health status, better quality of life and greater life expectancy (Avorn & Langer, 1982; Langer & Rodin, 1976; Rodin & Langer, 1977).

As the numbers of older persons, especially very old persons (beyond age 80), continue to increase, the amount of federal and state money available for health programs cannot keep pace with the growing need. Older persons are being discharged from hospitals more quickly, are being denied access to nursing homes in an increasing number of states, and are making do with home health care services that continue to meet only a small fraction of the growing need. In addition, there is less public funding for prevention and health promotion education through local health departments. Thus, in an era of reduced societal resources, illness prevention, health promotion, and self-care activities take on greater significance.

EXERCISE

Exercise refers to physical movements that are done on a regular basis to accomplish specific effects. Vigorous exercising, such as most aerobic dancing, is not necessary or perhaps wise for most elderly and, if done, should not be done every day. On the other hand, seniors who engage in mild once-a-week activities, as are available at many senior centers, are merely engaging in recreation, not exercise. Among these weekly participants, those who engage in vigorous activity tend to risk injury. The ideal exercise regimen for older persons is moderate exercise every other day or daily activity of a gentler nature.

A study of an exercise program for older persons residing at two senior centers reported that classes held three times a week were attended more conscientiously than weekly classes, despite the increased responsibility for attending classes (Haber, 1986a). Moreover, homework assignments were more conscientiously completed since the instructor could monitor "yesterday's" homework assignment, rather than the more vague "last week's" assignments. In addition, classes that met three times a week produced better health results, as expected, than classes that met weekly.

This study also compared yoga classes with mild aerobics for seniors and detected no differences between these types of classes. Both types of classes were regularly attended, and both produced better results when persons attended three times a week. The research design did not examine the range of physical benefits that could be attained through different interventions. Analysts have noted that different types of exercise programs are likely to produce results in specific areas (see Table 7.1).

Generally speaking, there are three types of exercise programs. The first set of programs is oriented to cardiovascular strengthening and increased endurance. Aerobic dance classes, brisk walks, bicycle rides, and swimming produce these benefits. Activities that allow gentle impact with the ground, like aerobic dance classes (preferably with wood floors and good sneakers) and brisk walks, may increase bone mineral content and stave off osteoporosis (Krolner et al., 1983; Smith, 1982). Fitness programs and exercising can impact on heart disease as well. Hodgson and Buskirk (1977) documented the positive impact of an exercise program on cardiovascular function in the elderly. DeVries (1970) and Sidney et al. (1977) report that regardless of the elderly person's prior exercise habits, an appropriate aerobic exercise program will increase maximum oxygen consumption between 10% and 30%. Studies of exercise programs with the elderly report decreases in systolic and diastolic blood pressure (Buccola & Stone, 1975; deVries, 1970; Haber, 1983c, 1986a).

Aerobic exercises are designed to stimulate the heart and lungs for a sufficient period of time (usually at least 20 to 25 minutes) to produce an increased and sustained target heart rate. The target heart rate is the optimal rate at which the heart should beat during exercise. As people age, the target heart rate declines. The heart, lungs, and circulatory system do not respond as well over the life cycle to the same stress level of exercise. Aerobic capacity (i.e., the ability of the cardiovascular system to transport oxygen to working muscles) declines every year after age 30. The heart muscle itself declines in contractibility. Thus, a vigorous walk for an elderly person can be roughly equivalent to serious jogging for a younger person.

For most older persons a target heart rate of 112 to 120 beats per minute is beneficial and safe. Those with heart disease, the very frail, or the very fit

TABLE 7.1 Exercise Activities and Fitness Components

Activities	Endurance	Strength	Flexibility	Balance	Coordination/ agility
Swimming	3[a]	3	3	3	3
Brisk walking (3.5–4 MPH)	3	2	1	1	1
Slow walking (2 MPH)	1	1	1	1	1
Calisthenics	1	1	2	2	2
Golf (walking)	1	2	2	2	2
Bowling	1	2	2	2	2
Tennis	2	2	2	2	2
Ballet	3	3	3	3	3
Rhythmic dancing	3	2	3	2	3
Yoga	1	1	3+	3+	2
Weight lifting[b]	0	3	0	2	1
Weight training	0	3	1	1	1
Cycling	3	3	3	3	3
Jogging, running	3	2	1	1	1
Football[c]	1–2	2–3	0	1	1–2
Baseball[c]	1	1	2	1	2
Basketball[c]	3	2	1	2	2
Soccer[c]	3	2	2	2	3

[a]Key: 3 = high level, 2 = moderate level, 1 = little effect, 0 = no appreciable effect.
[b]Can cause dangerous increases in blood pressure.
[c]Varies by position.
From Kuntzleman, C.T. (1978). *Rating the exercises*. New York: Penguin.

might want to alter this rate (see Table 7.2). To determine compliance with the target heart rate, individuals count their pulse beats for a 10-second period at periodic intervals, then multiply by six. An additional safety procedure uniformly followed by aerobics instructors is to provide a warm-up period and a cool-down phase before and after the target heart rate is achieved.

The essence of aerobic exercising is to engage in smooth, rhythmic, and continuous exercise, with a focus on the large muscles of the body. The primary health goals are to strengthen the cardiopulmonary system, prevent or postpone heart disease, energize the body, and improve psychological well-being. The most popular vehicles for aerobic exercising are brisk walks, which allow people to explore nature or people-watch, and aerobic dancing, which provides social opportunity and enjoyable music.

A second type of exercise program focuses on flexibility, balance, and relaxation. These programs are especially useful for those afflicted with arthritic aches and pains, the very frail (Haber, 1988b), and those recently discharged from a hospital, since the techniques are very gentle in their execution. Some persons supplement the cardiovascular benefits derived from an aerobic dance class, brisk walks, bicycling, or swimming with a flexibility, relaxation, or balance program such as yoga or Tai Chi.

Eastern traditions such as yoga and Tai Chi are ancient practices that the elderly can—and do—appreciate if separated from any type of religious commitment (Haber, 1979). The most widely practiced yoga in this country is hatha yoga, which is physical stretching, bending, and twisting, with an emphasis on relaxation and body awareness. Yoga is a noncompetitive discipline, with students working within their own capacity. Unlike many calisthenics courses where instructors exhort "no pain, no gain," yoga trainers advise "no strain, no pain." After body movements are completed, participants hold a posture for a brief time, while focusing on gentle breathing, body awareness, and relaxation.

The Easy Does It Yoga program is the most widely used yoga program for older persons in America (Christensen & Rankin, 1979). Instructors are trained to work with older persons, and the exercises are well within the limits of the participants. The first half of the course is designed for persons sitting in chairs. As students build up confidence and learn safety techniques for getting on and off the floor, there is a gradual move to include mat exercises as well.

All yoga courses include deep breathing (or yoga breaths) to utilize the entire lung capacity. This is a widely used stress management technique as well. Breathing deeply through the nose, individuals fill up their stomach first, then their chest, the reverse of what people typically mistake for deep breathing. (Ask people to take a deep breath and they typically expand their chest.) After a few minutes of practice most persons learn how to do belly breaths or, more technically, diaphragmatic breathing. For persons who are shallow breathers dizziness can occur after only two or three breaths. For most persons, however, the increased oxygenation of tissue produces an instant calming effect.

TABLE 7.2 Pulse Rate and Target Zone Chart

Age (years)	Target zone for heart beats during exercise (60–75% of maximum heart rate)	Average maximum heart rate (100%)
50	102–127 beats per minute	170
55	99–124 beats per minute	165
60	96–120 beats per minute	160
65	93–116 beats per minute	155
70	90–113 beats per minute	150
75	87–108 beats per minute	145
80	84–105 beats per minute	140
85	81–101 beats per minute	135
90	78–97 beats per minute	130

From National Heart, Lung, and Blood Institute. (1981). *Exercise and Your Heart* (NIH Publication No. 81-1677). Washington, DC: National Institutes of Health.

A third type of exercise program is weight lifting. As people age, the percentage of body fat, as opposed to lean muscle tissue, increases. Also occurring with age is the decline of general muscle strength. An appropriate weight lifting program, however, will improve muscle strength and endurance. It will help older persons who must carry heavy grocery bags to their cars and sometimes up steps to their front doors. In addition, household items get picked up or moved, jar lids need to be twisted off, and minor repairs have to be made. A good weight lifting class for seniors would not only be designed for the strength and endurance capacity of the older person, but would include safety tips on lifting objects and moving one's body to avoid muscle strain, backaches, hernias, and the like. While there are few weight lifting programs available to older persons, weight lifting components are increasingly being incorporated into the more popular aerobic classes.

All three types of exercise programs should be preceded by a complete physical examination at the doctor's office. Since some physicians are not especially health conscious, care should be taken to select a person who recognizes the importance of exercise for seniors. Even today there are probably health care professionals who subscribe to the old wives' tale that exercise is not good for older persons, it is too taxing, and at a certain point in life it is unnecessary.

Access is also a major consideration for starting exercise programs. One reason brisk walks are the most popular form of exercise is that they do not cost anything. You can begin as soon as you leave your front door and equipment is not needed. You do not have to wait for available space or for other persons (unless you choose the company). Also, you can vary the monotony by walking in different directions to observe new things in nature or to find new people to watch.

While walking is perhaps the most accessible form of exercise, other forms of exercise are becoming more convenient. An increasing variety of courses is springing up at senior centers, YMCAs, YWCAs, city recreation departments, community centers, hospital health promotion programs, universities or community colleges, public schools, and health associations. Information and referral are provided by the local area agency on aging, the local chapter of the American Association of Retired Persons, neighborhood schools, community colleges or universities, public health departments, and for special health problems, like arthritis, heart disease, and cancer, their local foundations or associations.

Finally, health promotion programs that are initially dependent on professional expertise and grant funding should incorporate a peer leadership or self-help component (Haber, 1986a). In this way occasional consultation with professionals can take the place of ongoing dependency. In addition to professional consultation, educational materials can help older persons become more knowledgeable about their exercise programs, more independent, and better teachers for their peers.

NUTRITION EDUCATION

Nutrition is the science that deals with the effect of food on health and disease. Nutrition education is the application of healthful eating habits to one's own diet. The basic components of nutrition education are obtaining an appropriate amount of calories to maintain/attain optimal body weight; eating a variety of fresh fruits and vegetables, complex carbohydrates, lean meats, and low-fat dairy products; eliminating excess salt, sugar, fats, and alcohol; acquiring sufficient water and fiber; and obtaining adequate nutrient intake or supplements appropriate to one's physical condition and drug therapy (Nestle, 1983).

The major obstacles to achieving this well-balanced diet for older persons are the three *m*'s—malnutrition, metabolism, and medications.

1. Malnutrition: Inadequate nutrient intake occurs among the elderly for a variety of reasons. First, reduced appetite is often a consequence of eating alone. The rationale for the congregate meal programs funded through the Older Americans Act is to provide the companionship necessary for many persons who are used to eating as part of a family but no longer do so. Second, elders who eat alone are also handicapped by food manufacturers who do not produce nourishing food in small portions. Campbell's low-sodium single serving soups have been a step in the right direction. Third, malnutrition occurs for many older persons who are on fixed incomes. Deficient nutrient intake is more evident among the poor elderly (Lowenstein, 1982). One way to cut corners, for instance, is to obtain 1- or 2-day-old food that has been discounted, but has also lost much of its nutritional value. Fourth, limited physical capacity or mobility can affect one's ability to shop for food or to prepare meals. Fifth, ill-fitting dentures—or the lack of such—can make the act of eating uncomfortable.

2. Metabolism: The basal metabolic rate, which reflects the energy level of the body, declines about 20% from age 20 to age 70. Thus, the amount of calories needed declines steadily with age as well. Those who do not reduce caloric intake between the ages of 45 and 70 are likely to gain weight, and obesity is a factor in contracting or worsening chronic diseases. Those who do reduce caloric intake must guard against the loss of essential vitamins, minerals, and protein. Food chosen in late life, therefore, must be calorie poor but nutrient rich. Acknowledging that the new generation of retirees may be more calorie conscious, the Central Missouri Area Agency on Aging offers a low-calorie alternative menu at its congregate meal site for older adults.

3. Medications: Many of the most common problems with aging—constipation, insomnia, arthritic aches and pains, hypertension, and the like—can be altered through diet. The alternative of choice for many persons, however, is medication. Many drugs, like laxatives and sleeping pills, lose their effectiveness in a short while. Moreover, drugs can also produce harmful side effects.

Several popular techniques are used in most nutrition education courses. Keeping a journal is the easiest way to become more aware of what you eat and shouldn't, as well as what you don't eat and should. Going one step further, persons can count the calories in their journal to achieve the desired number that maintains optimal weight. In addition to counting calories in foods, calories expended through exercises and activities can also be counted during the course of the day. A record of calories burned is helpful in determining the number of calories that can be consumed.

Most nutrition education courses provide healthful recipes for students and suggest healthy ways to prepare foods. Serious students will then make an easy-to-use filing system for their recipes. The filing system may also include foods for special diets, such as high-fiber, low-salt, low-fat, low-cholesterol, low-sugar, or low-caffeine diets.

Additional courses, books, and other modes of education and information can be accessed through contact with public health departments, heart/diabetes/cancer and other health associations, nutritional organizations, health food stores, the U.S. Department of Agriculture, the local American Association of Retired Persons chapter, and other community organizations and agencies that provide literature, seminars, workshops, and classes.

STRESS MANAGEMENT

Stress is a stimulus that demands a response on the part of an individual. The stress response is a general physiological response to an event, such as anxiety, fear, irritability, or excitement. Regardless of whether the stimulus is perceived to be positive or negative, the physiological response to stressful events will produce an increased pulse rate, blood pressure level, and respiratory rate; the release of hormones; vascular constriction and muscular tension; gastrointestinal distress; and an activation of the liver and spleen (Selye, 1976).

In the early stage of human history the cave dwellers' typical response to stress was to fight or flee. In contemporary America these two responses are often inappropriate. We must learn how to flow as well. *Stress management* refers to a variety of basic relaxation techniques to enhance the individual's capacity to cope with stressful events. Typically thought of as a tool for college students and business executives, stress management is most appropriate for older persons as well. Along with age comes an increased vulnerability to substantial amounts of stressful changes, such as the death of a spouse or other close family members, retirement and changes in financial status, vulnerability to institutionalization, failing eyesight or hearing and other health problems, losing a driver's license, limits on mobility, and engaging in a radically different set of responsibilities.

Stress is not limited to unpleasant events. Weddings, the birth of grandchildren and great grandchildren, the job promotion of an adult child and the subsequent geographical mobility, holidays and dates that remind one of significant past events or relationships, and the long anticipated retirement and moving to a desirable retirement community are also stressors on the body and mind. Holmes and Masuda (1973) demonstrated a correlation between the frequency and intensity of positive and negative major life events and the onset of psychiatric or medical diseases. These major life events were modified by Amster and Krauss (1974) into a geriatric social readjustment questionnaire appropriate to persons age 70 and above. While not statistically conclusive, the frequency and intensity of major life events in old age were related to mental and physical breakdown.

A wide variety of stress management techniques have been applied to young and old alike, including Hatha yoga, deep breathing, positive thinking, and biofeedback. Three of the most commonly employed techniques are progressive relaxation, visualization, and meditation.

1. Progressive relaxation: Progressive relaxation is a technique of tensing and relaxing muscle groups in a systematic way (Jacobson, 1938, 1962). In brief, participants progressively focus on specific parts of the body, beginning with the head (scalp, forehead, jaw, etc.) and ending with the foot (ankles, arches, toes). Different practitioners employ varying styles of relaxation, such as stressing the feeling of heaviness or warmth in each body part, imagining the relaxation of tension from each part, or merely tensing and relaxing each part.

2. Visualization: The serious student of stress management will allow 20 to 25 minutes for progressive relaxation, and then follow it with an equal period of time for visualization. Two popular variants of the visualization technique are to imagine a diseased part of the body healing itself and to imagine visiting a beautiful natural setting and interacting with a wise person (perhaps a deceased parent or grandparent who was greatly respected), who helps solve a problem.

3. Meditation: Unlike the other two techniques, meditation is rarely done in a prone position because of the ease with which it can transform itself into a nap. While a nap is not necessarily a poor form of stress management, meditation has been associated with an even deeper physiological state of relaxation than sleep (Wallace, 1970). Sitting comfortably (for most older persons this does not mean the lotus position) with arms and legs uncrossed, the person gently focuses on a nonsense syllable, a mantra (a sound with an alleged spiritual quality), a word, or a phrase (Benson, 1976) and repeats it silently, easily, and gently. When thoughts intrude on the repetition of the sound, the person gently detaches himself or herself from these thoughts and returns to the meditative sound. The quantity of thoughts intruding on a meditation is unrelated to the effect of the meditation.

Stress management techniques are deceptively simple. They are deceptive in the sense that while they are easy and enjoyable to learn, it is difficult to sustain a new daily habit. It may be useful to have a partner or to be part of a group of friends who can encourage each other to persist. Also, it is important to establish a consistent routine, such as just before breakfast and dinner, to form a daily habit.

There are many other avenues to stress management, such as exercise, diet, spiritual development, hobbies, recreation, and social support, to name a few. The popular methods of stress management just described, however, tend to help people become aware of their own physical and mental responses to stress. By understanding how stress impacts on one's own body and mind, one may attain an even deeper relaxation level, which will help to restore the body to a healthful state.

WELLNESS PROGRAMS

For many years comprehensive illness centers (hospitals, nursing homes, and medical clinics) have been available to sick or injured persons. Recently the comprehensive wellness center has taken its place alongside these more traditional health facilities. Many of these centers cater to the needs of aging persons. They can be located in any type of facility and offer a unique range of services.

Hospitals, for example, are opening wellness centers as the amount of occupied bed space declines. St. Vincent Hospital and Health Care Center in Indianapolis opened in 1979 and set aside almost 9,000 square feet of space for classrooms, a gymnasium, and staff offices. In one class, called Body Recall, students with an average age of 82 years enjoyed performing muscle-toning exercises to music. Exercise courses were supplemented with health education sessions on such topics as nutrition, cardiopulmonary resuscitation, wellness assessment, smoking cessation, and so forth. A similar program was offered at the Ohio Presbyterian Homes throughout the state (Slivinske & Kosberg, 1984), with enrollees (average age 76) participating in education, physical exercises, and counseling as part of the Personal Health Management System program. Another program attracted 30% of 300 residents in a life care facility in Alexandria, Virginia. Older persons participated in a wellness program conducted by two gerontological nurses (Barbaro & Noyes, 1984).

Several wellness centers offer comprehensive health promotion opportunities for older persons. The original prototype began in northern California in the early 1970s, through the Senior Actualization Growth Exploration (SAGE) program. Older students with higher than average educational and income levels joined physical exercise classes, biofeedback and other stress management techniques, group therapy or encounter groups, yoga, Tai Chi, and a range of innovative techniques that heretofore were only experimented with by the young.

Two of the most comprehensive wellness programs began in the late 1970s in Seattle, Washington, and Santa Monica, California. The Wallingford Wellness Project was originally funded by the Administration on Aging and in 1979 implemented by the School of Social Work at the University of Washington and Senior Services and Centers of King County, Washington. One of the original programs took place at a senior center and offered participants physical fitness classes, nutrition education, stress management techniques, and personal and community self-help ideas and techniques. This latter component included advocacy activities for a better community and society—a political component that is missing from most health promotion programs (Minkler, 1983). While the program is intergenerational, three fourths of the participants were over age 60 and the oldest was 84. Several years later, the program continues in other forms, including the vehicle of self-help groups that are organized and implemented by seniors who graduated from one of the original programs.

The program in Santa Monica, California, was titled the Healthy Lifestyle for Seniors Project (Fallcreek & Stam, 1982). It began in 1978 and has been replicated in Arizona and New York. The program was initiated at several sites around Santa Monica, including a senior center, a YWCA, a government subsidized housing project, a retirement home, and a VA hospital. The project offered older persons classes on health monitoring, nutrition, exercise, and stress management, and it was subsidized by the Meals for Millions/Freedom from Hunger Foundation.

SELF-CARE

Self-care is "a process whereby a lay person can function effectively on his or her own behalf in health promotion and decision-making, in disease prevention, detection, and treatment at the level of the primary health resource in the health care system" (Levin, 1986). Taking care of one's own health has been a primary modus operandi for people throughout recorded history. Our pioneer forefathers had to be rugged individualists, skeptical of authority. Over the 20th century, however, we have increasingly relied on experts, or specialists, especially in the area of health care. Today the majority of the problems that send us to doctors are or could be self-correcting. In the absence of knowing when a symptom or behavior change is a serious health problem masquerading as a minor ailment, we rely on experts for our health care needs.

T. Franklin Williams, director of the National Institute on Aging, commented on the need for more self-care programs (one of which is currently being developed and evaluated by the American Association of Retired Persons) as follows:

> *[This program] is by no means meant [to be] a substitute for medical care. It is, however, a way to promote awareness, encourage a healthier lifestyle, and offer constructive suggestions to an individual responsible for his or her own health management. It is meant as a guide that should help people become knowledge-*

*able about the body in the hope of avoiding some detrimental habits and adopting some that may be beneficial toward a healthy old age. (Nelson et al., 1986)**

In an era of health care cost containment, older persons and their family caregivers must assume greater responsibility for monitoring health in the home setting. Older persons are being discharged earlier from hospitals and are increasingly denied access to nursing home care. At the same time, resources for home- and community-based alternatives are not increasing fast enough to meet the need. It is most useful, therefore, for elders and their informal caregivers to learn the skills and information needed to maintain independence in the home setting. The utility of such learning is heightened by two facts: (1) Almost 90% of the elderly are coping with a chronic condition and (2) chronic care in the community is not reimbursable through Medicare.

Some of the more useful self-care skills that need to be learned are taking blood pressure; performing CPR, the Heimlich maneuver, and first aid; reading a thermometer; taking a pulse; and accessing free or low-cost community resources (medical screenings, Alcoholics Anonymous, smoking cessation programs, etc.). Another component of self-care is the ability to manage the complexity of the drug regimens that many older persons must contend with. Drug management includes such activities as being alerted to the way medications interact with each other, as well as with food, beverages, and supplements; remembering multiple medication schedules; and being cautious about the long-term use of medications. While most drug research is not conducted over a 20- to 30-year period, older persons may be taking medication this long. Other important components of a self-care program are recognizing the signs and symptoms of disease; practicing self-care hygiene; maintaining one's own program of stress reduction, nutrition, or exercise; playing a more active role when interacting with health professionals and using the medical care system; and identifying appropriate associations and self-help groups for support and continuing education.

As medical science and technology develop into a sophisticated system of health care, individual responsibility for care is replaced with a passive reliance on physicians and other health professionals. People increasingly assume that advanced scientific knowledge and technological procedures are more effective than "home remedies." At the same time, however, individual autonomy is gradually relinquished to the bureaucratic demands of care in an institution such as a clinic, hospital, or nursing home. Not surprisingly, distrust and dissatisfaction have increased as the health care system becomes more responsive to institutional needs and less responsive to individual needs.

Self-care has a strong prevention and promotion facet to it that has been increasingly sought by health consumers but has not yet been widely adopted by the traditional medical community. Since the 1970s, several dozen medical self-care manuals have been published to help people measure their own blood pressure levels, count pulse rates, take temperatures, check for swollen glands and sore throats, and so on. Many self-care initiatives have become widely practiced and habitual, including monthly breast examinations, home medical tests to identify disease or pregnancy, cardiopulmonary resuscitation, the Heimlich method, home safety techniques, assertiveness training, weight loss programs, smoking cessation techniques, food cooperatives, and self-help groups for specific health problems.

Self-care goes beyond the traditional goal of patient education. It is a comprehensive strategy to encourage persons to care for themselves through a program of disease prevention, health promotion, and the diagnosis and treatment of illness. In this latter regard, persons are taught to think systematically about which problems can be cared for without professional assistance and when such assistance is required. At least 75% of health care is self-care (Williamson & Danaher, 1978) and includes activities that both substitute for and supplement professional intervention (Steiger & Lipson, 1985). The essence of self-care activity is the emphasis on personal responsibility for achieving wellness and managing disease. This responsibility involves learning health care skills, taking the initiative in selecting educational materials, and taking an active role in health care decisionmaking.

The growth of the self-care movement is evidenced by the accelerating number of publications, conferences, and classes that have been initiated in the past decade. In part this growth can be attributed to a shift in major health problems from acute to chronic conditions. Chronic conditions are not cured; they are coped with. They require ongoing, multifaceted support, the kind that health care professionals do not provide and that most health consumers will need to do as much as possible on their own. In this era of health care cost containment, the scope of professional or paraprofessional care for chronic conditions that will be subsidized through government or private insurance programs will be severely limited. Aside from cost, it is useful for older persons and their caregivers to monitor their health condition on an ongoing basis rather than rely on infrequent professional contact. The diagnosis of a medical problem by a health care professional is enhanced if the older person or family caregiver has monitored the course of a chronic condition between visits.

Monitoring medications is also an important component of self-care. While the elderly constitute 12% of the population, they consume almost 30% of the nation's prescribed and over-the-counter medications. Given the multiplicity of doctors and pharmacists used by the elderly, combined with unregulated over-the-counter use of medications, it is the responsibility of older persons or family caregivers to keep a comprehensive list of all medications taken and to routinely inform pharmacists and doctors as they fill prescriptions or prescribe medications. Individuals must also be alert for the opportunity to reduce medication usage and to take the initiative in suggesting this to their physicians, especially when diet and exercise routines have been implemented and are having an impact on health.

Ultimately, compliance with medication schedules is in the hands of older persons and their caregivers. Consumers must read labels carefully, know when drugs should be taken during the course of the day, keep themselves informed about new medications entering the market, heed existing written cautions on packaging or package inserts (as well as be alert to the latest warnings that may appear through the media), and seek new packaging or memory devices that facilitate compliance to schedules.

Another important technique for self-care is to access different sources of information on the same health topic to be aware of conflicting opinions. The professional then becomes a collaborator in health care, not merely an authoritarian figure giving orders to a passive patient. To accomplish this, one can join self-help groups or health associations, take courses, and attend seminars or workshops. Some who practice self-care become health advocates devoting considerable time to informing others of health care alternatives, lobbying legislators, or joining their local Gray Panther chapters or other advocacy organizations in their community. Self-care advocates are not medically trained to make decisions independently for themselves or others, but they do have an obligation to widen the knowledge base of each individual who is attempting to find the best health care in an increasingly complex and varied health care system.

SELF-CARE PROGRAMS

One model of a self-care program is the Dartmouth Self-Care for Senior Citizens Program (Simmons et al., 1986). Based at Dartmouth's medical school in Hanover, New Hampshire, the program has educated several hundred older persons in medical self-care, illness prevention, and the effective use of health and social services. The course content is divided into three segments:

1. Medical care: Acquiring access to the medical care system, learning medical self-care skills, and correctly utilizing the medical care system
2. Life-style: Assuming responsibility for one's own welfare (e.g., physical fitness, emotional well-being, dietary patterns)
3. Independent living: Being aware of the social services available in the community and having the ability to use such agencies (Simmons et al., 1986)

Data from the Dartmouth program's research project revealed that self-care graduates, in comparison to a control group, had improved health knowledge and continued to improve after a 1-year follow-up; expressed more confidence in their performance of self-care skills and demonstrated their ability to perform these skills; expressed a belief they could communicate more effectively with their personal physician; used self-care books to cope with health problems; engaged in multiple attempts to change health habits (exercise, nutrition, weight control, stress management); and reported improved mental health.

The American Association of Retired Persons is currently testing a similar self-care program for seniors (Kane-Williams et al., 1986; Nelson et al., 1986). The 11-week course has a medical and a life-style section. The class content for the medical section is as follows:*

1. Health care: Whose responsibility?
   Skill: Read a thermometer
2. Selected health situations: How to identify and manage
   Skill: First aid for choking
3. Medications: What you need to know
   Skill: Fill out a medication record
4. Common health problems: Causes, symptoms, and treatments
   Skill: Take a resting pulse
5. More common health problems: Causes, symptoms, and treatments
   Skill: Take a blood pressure reading

The life-style section covers the following:*

6. Life-styles: Taking action to promote health
   Skill: Blood pressure review
7. Exercise: Getting fit and feeling fine
   Skill: Take an exercise heart rate or pulse
8. Nutrition: Eating to stay healthy
   Skill: Nutritious meal planning
9. Emotional well-being: It's your world
   Skill: Progressive muscle relaxation technique
10. Consumer issues in health care
    Skill: Use the directory of local human and social service agencies
11. Self-change plan: Planning a better tomorrow
    Skill: Design a self-change plan

The most innovative aspect of this program is its workbook, which can allow both the participant and the researcher to measure changes in knowledge, attitude, skills, and utilization patterns (Kane-Williams et al., 1986). The evaluation of this program was still in progress in 1988.

The Healthwise project in Boise, Idaho, devotes some of its time to promoting two handbooks for older adults: *Growing Younger Handbook* (Kemper,

D., et al., 1987) and *Growing Wiser: The Older Person's Guide to Mental Wellness* (Kemper et al., 1986). The *Growing Younger Handbook* is primarily a self-care manual that examines principles of self-care, describes self-care techniques, and discusses ways to prevent, recognize, and treat common illnesses. There are additional sections on how to interact with health care professionals, negotiate with health care bureaucracies, maintain health records, and get the most from exercise, relaxation, and nutrition activities.

Growing Wiser focuses on memory, mental alertness, communication, and other aspects of mental health. On almost every page is a pithy saying or quotation. In the chapter on mental alertness the authors provide the following rule of thumb: "If you go to a store and forget what you came to buy, it's of little mental concern—next time bring a list. If you forget what you are supposed to do in the store—that's serious." While the emphasis is on readability, the content of both handbooks has been developed in concert with a wide variety of health and medical experts. For those who cannot be motivated no matter how readable the reading matter, Healthwise provides neighborhood-based health promotion workshop programs for older adults, which attempt to reinforce the concepts and practices described in the handbooks.

A pretest-posttest evaluation of the 8-hour Growing Wiser Workshop program was completed in January 1987. Statistical findings on almost 600 older Boise, Idaho, residents reveal that participants had improved on a geriatric depression scale and on a name-face memory test (Kemper, 1987). An earlier evaluation of the Growing Younger program reported statistically significant positive changes in fitness levels, eating and drinking behaviors, stress management, social interaction, and medical care behaviors (Kemper, 1984).

The Wisdom project is a self-care program sponsored by the American Red Cross in greater New York. It teaches older adults to recognize the signs and symptoms of disease, to maintain their own program of stress reduction, nutrition, and exercise, and to play a more active role when using the medical care system (Lederman et al., 1983). Yet another medical self-care system trains older persons to periodically and systematically assess bodily symptoms for onset, location, duration, character, course, associated symptoms, aggravated factors, relieving factors, and previous treatments (Warner-Reitz, 1981). Many of these older persons are using self-scoring tests to assess their risk for the number one and three killers in America—heart attack and stroke.

8

SELF-HELP GROUPS

WHAT ARE SELF-HELP GROUPS?

Simply stated, self-help groups are associations of people who come together to share a similar concern for the purpose of mutual support. These groups are substantially different from conventional health and social service agencies, where professionals and administrators define client needs, determine services, and establish goals. Instead, groups are peer-controlled or egalitarian organizations, which emphasize personal responsibility within a context of interdependence. The purposes of group meetings are to share accounts of similar experiences and foster mutual support, to compare and develop attitudinal and behavioral coping strategies, and to identify and gain access to services and resources. Typically the groups are small, informal, and meet on a regular basis.

Self-help groups have become the single largest source of support in America during the past decade. Joiners have surpassed the numbers of persons who seek assistance from mental health professionals or from clergy (Mellinger & Balter, 1983). The likely explanation for this growth is the unique set of strengths associated with self-help groups in a cost containment era. One such strength of the self-help movement is its potential for *empowerment.* In a world where people feel little power to resolve larger issues such as budget deficits and nuclear stockpiling and in a society where people must contend with increasingly bureaucratized and computerized organizations, there is an opportunity at the neighborhood level to make active, positive, and personal advancement toward coping with a problem in a fiscally responsible way. Self-help participants are empowered in a number of ways: through the process of volunteering to join, the willingness to share in leadership functions, the capacity to take a positive attitude toward adversity, the desire to engage in mutually reinforcing activities, and the interest in advocating on behalf of a cause larger than oneself.

In contrast to these activities, other types of assistance that people seek for mental or physical health problems typically entail waiting for appointments; passively receiving guidance; conforming to time limits, fee schedules, and other constraints to service; and coping with the perceived stigma (especially among older persons) of seeking help from mental health professionals.

Empowerment can be achieved not only on an individual or small group level, but at the community or societal level as well. Regarding community network building, for instance, Hess (1982) notes that the self-help movement is

> *a movement away from an over-reliance on professionals in an increasingly professionalized society toward the concept of neighbor helping neighbor and friend helping friend. It builds enduring relationships among people so that they may assist each other in areas far beyond those that originally brought them together. Self-help may conserve resources, such as energy and professionals, but its greatest promise lies in the building of these enduring relationships, for they are the foundation of strong, supportive, and lasting communities. (pp. 1–2)**

At the societal level, local self-help groups have banded together to change institutions through developing or modifying state and federal regulations and legislation. One example among many that can be offered, is the advocacy efforts of the support group, Friends and Relatives of the Institutionalized Aged (FRIA), which began in 1976 in New York City under the leadership of Dr. Rose Dobrof. While some local FRIA groups met only to share their personal concerns and coping strategies, others were actively forming nationwide alliances to change regulations regarding nursing home care standards (National Council on the Aging, 1982). These FRIA groups have blocked the New York State Health Department's attempt to relax standards for nursing home care and pressured the New York State Department of Social Services into revising regulations to allow more residents access to their nursing home beds after being hospitalized.

A second unique aspect of self-help groups is *accessibility,* in every aspect of the word. Self-help group members are accessible to each other in emergencies and over prolonged periods of time (which is crucial considering the preponderance of chronic conditions that afflict the nation's aging). Members can also help prevent emergencies before they arise. Because they are self-help groups their members have access to this help without exorbitant charges, bureaucratic forms, appointment times, transportation out of the neighborhood,

*Copyright 1982 by Haworth Press. Reprinted with permission.

impersonal officials, or unresponsive regulations. Moreover, federal and state policy decisions that limit spending on human services do not limit the accessibility of self-help groups. In fact, they make these groups even more vital during the current era of austerity and future vicissitudes of public funding.

A third unique feature of the self-help group is its emphasis on *experiential* insight, or specialized information about a problem based on personal experience (Borkman, 1982). Experiential knowledge is a two-stage process: (1) to reflect on the validity of one's own experiences and those of others in similar situations through the sharing of information and (2) to attempt new ideas and behaviors to cope with challenges in everyday life. This process allows individuals to select and validate information gathered from the collective experiences of other group members. Often a modeling process is evident, whereby an individual who has successfully coped with an earlier developmental challenge is able to provide insight to other persons who are approaching or are in the midst of this problem. Experiential knowledge involves disclosure and caring about people rather than health problems or conditions. Practical information is gained through offering and receiving ideas in a unique and spontaneous fashion.

It is not just empowerment, accessibility, and experiential insight that draw people to the self-help group movement, but the era in which we live. Over the past few decades we have borne the brunt of increasing mobility: job transfers, urban redevelopment, retirement relocation, and other factors that contribute to family, friends, and neighbors coping with dwindling neighborhood support networks. Exacerbating this mobility problem is the continuing decline of birthrates, which has started to limit the number of children and grandchildren who are important components of informal networks. When these eroding supports are combined with decreasing resources at human service agencies, the result is a growing demand for self-help knowledge and accessible mutual aid. Thus, the growth of self-help groups is a response to the times.

Finally, while self-help groups are primarily peer oriented, the potential for professional impact is substantial. Support group members can apply their increasing experience and skill at expressing themselves with peers and in their dealings with professionals as well. They can share their insights on coping with illness, from both an attitudinal and a practical management perspective, as well as bring neglected problem areas to the attention of professionals and students. One example of peer contribution to professional development was a visit made by representatives from a self-help group to a medical school in order to sensitize medical students to their efforts at coping with a specific illness (Madara, 1986).

Another avenue for wider impact is the transformation of local self-help groups into national health associations and foundations. Numerous examples of this can be cited, including Alcoholics Anonymous; American Association of

Retired Persons' Widowed Persons Services; United Cerebral Palsy Association; National Association of Retarded Citizens; Parents Anonymous; Lupus Foundation; Multiple Sclerosis Society; Committee to Combat Huntington's Disease; Recovery, Inc.; and Compassionate Friends. Other self-help groups enhance their impact by affiliating with national associations, such as Mended Hearts and stroke clubs within the American Heart Association, arthritis groups within the Arthritis Foundation, and Reach to Recovery within the American Cancer Society.

Whether it is at the local or national level, self-help group members typically advocate for tearing down stereotypes and stigmas associated with specific health conditions and for implementing more responsive government legislation. These public education goals are furthered through lobbying efforts such as letter-writing campaigns, conferences, media presentations, fund raising, demonstrations, and boycotts. Often these efforts begin at the local level, through group members sharing unfulfilled needs or encountering negative attitudes and restrictive or nonexistent legislation. As group members begin to empower each other, the eventual outcomes can have broad societal ramifications.

HOW PERVASIVE ARE THEY?

By almost any measure of growth, the self-help group movement is a phenomenon to be reckoned with. By 1979 participants in such groups had expanded to 15 million people and 500,000 different groups (Evans, 1979). These 1979 estimates are now too conservative, given the documented growth among groups by self-help clearinghouses over the past several years. By 1983 self-help groups were the number one source of assistance to persons with mental health problems. A probability sample of over 3,000 households revealed that more individuals used self-help groups (5.8%) than sought help from mental health professionals (5.6%) or consulted with clergy or pastoral sources (5%) (Mellinger & Balter, 1983). Yet another indicator of growth is the number of state and area self-help clearinghouses (i.e., referral and networking centers), which increased almost 50% in less than 5 years, from 20 in mid-1981 to 29 in early 1986.

Two of the most successful clearinghouses, at Denville, New Jersey, and Evanston, Illinois, have documented a dramatic growth in telephone referrals to existing groups, and in the development of new groups. Shortly after beginning operations both centers logged hundreds of calls for referrals. Innumerable requests for information were received as well. In terms of self-help group development, the New Jersey center developed more than 100 new groups the first year (1981) alone. From 1981 to 1983 the number of self-help groups identified in New Jersey went from 70 to 3,200—all of which were listed in an easily accessible data base.

The surgeon general's report on health promotion (*Healthy people,* 1979) confirmed that the self-help movement constituted a significant community resource and the rapid growth of self-help groups attested to their ability to meet social needs that could not be filled by family, voluntary community organizations, or health agencies alone. Another government report from the U.S. Department of Health and Human Services (Office of Human Development Services, 1984) recommended that the number of persons served by such groups should be doubled during the 1980s. This contention was supported by a study in California, which revealed that while 75% of the respondents to a survey agreed that "when facing a life crisis, it would be useful to talk to someone else who had been through a similar situation," only 9% of adults actually did consult with someone about the same problem (Department of Mental Health, 1979). According to Ed Madara, director of the New Jersey Self Help Clearinghouse "the full potential of utilizing self-help groups remains untapped" (1986).

Budgetary constraints and modest economic growth will limit the service capability of human service agencies and the availability of professional assistance. Thus, self-help groups have the potential for considerable additional growth. This opinion is supported by futurists as well. John Naisbitt reported in *Megatrends* (1982) that the major shift from institutional help to self-help/mutual aid is one of the 10 major trends transforming American Society. Alvin Toffler in *The Third Wave* (1980) cited self-help groups as one of the dominant forces for change in American society and an influence that is likely to accelerate in its growth.

AGE-RELATED SELF-HELP GROUPS

The involvement of aging persons in self-help groups is widely discussed in the literature (Borkman, 1982; Haber, 1983b, 1984b; Lieberman, 1985; Riessman et al., 1984; Riessman & Moody, 1982). While the discussion has been far ranging, two consistent observations frequently appear. First, there is substantial evidence that this type of support group is especially appropriate for the chronic care needs of aging persons and their caregivers. Second, the number of aging persons and their caregivers in self-help groups is growing, and there is great potential for an even faster growth rate.

The appropriateness of self-help groups for aging persons and their caregivers is based on a number of converging factors. One such factor is the declining number of natural supports available to present and future cohorts of elderly. Declining birthrates, for instance, mean fewer children and grandchildren as caregiving resources. Also job mobility, retirement relocation, and neighborhood growth or renewal often result in the dispersion of family, friends, and neighbors who assist the aging with informal support. At the same time, the elderly are often afflicted with mobility limitations due to health factors or unwillingness to travel out of their own neighborhood and are more dependent on informal support in the immediate neighborhood.

Another factor that contributes to the relevance of self-help groups is the elderly person's reluctance to use mental health professionals. Butler and Lewis (1982) note some of the barriers on the part of the elderly themselves, such as the perceived stigma in seeking out professional assistance and the reluctance to seek assistance within a large, impersonal, and highly bureaucratic organizational structure. In addition, there is a reluctance on the part of many health professionals who perceive mental health problems as irreversible in old age. Other professionals do not want to cope with Medicare paperwork and regulations as well as seek the additional reimbursement from the older client who is not covered by insurance.

Yet another factor that indicates how appropriate self-help groups can be for older persons is the chronic nature of the health problems of the elderly. Eighty-seven percent of older persons are afflicted with one or more chronic health conditions that demand long-term rehabilitation or coping strategies, including the management of complex medication schedules. Many of these persons with chronic conditions are dependent on informal caregivers, a substantial number of whom are elderly themselves. These caregivers must contend with cumulative problems often without training, adequate respite, or information on how to access necessary support. Thus, it is not surprising that one of the fastest growing support groups at the present time is for caregivers of the elderly. Some of these groups focus on general problems associated with caregiving, while others are focused on the specific problems of caring for Alzheimer's patients (Clark & Rakowski, 1983; Riessman & Moody, 1982) or stroke victims (McCarthy, 1980; Riessman et al., 1984).

While the number of old people and family caregivers in self-help groups is growing, the precise figures on this growth are vague given the limited number of empirical studies that have been conducted (Butler et al., 1979). One indication that this growth is taking place, however, is the wide range of age-related health conditions (e.g., Alzheimer's disease, arthritis, emphysema, heart disease, cancer, and stroke) newly served by self-help groups (Borkman, 1982; Riessman et al., 1984). The evidence indicates that these types of support groups have age distributions similar to the general population affiliated with these health conditions (i.e., a disproportionate number of persons age 50 or over). Other new groups are developing around age-related conditions that attract older persons in proportions *less* than expected (based on the demographics of those afflicted in the general population); nevertheless, these groups are considerable in absolute numbers.

Lieberman and Borman (1979), for instance, note that while the percentage of widows over 60 in the general population is about 50%, widows over 60 represent only 20% of those who join widowhood groups nationwide. Nonetheless, 20% of existing membership does constitute a substantial number of elderly in support groups. Moreover, under the leadership of the AARP's Widowed Persons Service (WPS), the number of older widows who will become support group members is likely to increase. A study by Prisuta (1984) reported that WPS served about 25,000 of the estimated 1,200,000 persons who became widowed in 1983. The same principle holds true for Mended Hearts, a group dealing with the aftermath of heart surgery. Lieberman (1985) reports that while the percentage of persons age 60 and over in these groups is underrepresented when compared to the general population with heart surgery, they still constitute a substantial 40% of current self-help group membership.

Given the number of chronic conditions that disproportionately affect those age 60 and above in the population, the rate of membership growth in self-help groups by older persons and their caregivers has great potential. A partial list of these health conditions that disproportionately affect older persons and could lead to a future surge in self-help group membership includes arthritis, osteoporosis, hearing and visual impairment, late onset diabetes, heart disease, hypertension, Alzheimer's disease, ostomies, laryngectomies, stroke, cancer, Parkinson's disease, incontinence, medication compliance, sleep disorder, depression, caregiving for terminal illness, bereavement, and pulmonary disease.

There are additional reasons that the incidence of age-related self-help groups may accelerate. Hospitals, for instance, are feeling the pressure to speed up the discharge process due to Medicare's prospective payment system. Discharge social workers are concerned, however, about releasing patients whose caregivers may be overwhelmed by the tasks involved. Since 75% of patients treated in hospitals are suffering from chronic conditions that require ongoing help from caregivers in the community, the potential for additional group formation is great (Borman, 1983). Thus, hospitals have the potential for systematically implementing training programs for the caregivers of the elderly as part of the discharge procedure (Madara & Neigher, 1986).

Another factor that can stimulate the growth of age-related self-help groups is professional education. Borkman (1982) reviewed the literature on the aging, for example, and concluded that gerontologists were woefully ignorant of the purpose and function of self-help groups. Toseland (1985) and Toseland and Hacker (1982) examined the knowledge of self-help groups by social work practitioners and concluded that much education is needed by these professionals, especially since many are likely to be involved in support group formation or maintenance. If these educational gaps are filled, the potential for self-help/mutual aid development will accelerate.

Another barrier to the growth of age-related groups is that there are no clearinghouses for information focused on the problems of the aging. An examination of several state and regional self-help clearinghouse directories reveals that many existing age-related self-help groups have not been identified, thus suppressing their potential for growth.

A final consideration in the growth of age-related self-help groups is the potential to develop second-generation groups for older persons or their caregivers. Borkman (1982) notes, for example, that some existing support groups for alcoholics are youth oriented and, in fact, ignore a major ageism problem among the staff at treatment centers. The young staff members in two such groups regarded the older alcoholics as incurable and used language that the older persons found offensive. Thus, two second-generation groups for older alcoholics were begun to reduce the impact of ageism on the recidivism rates of older alcoholics. Both support groups led to better recovery rates among older alcoholics and increased the potential for working successfully with more older persons.

COLLABORATION BETWEEN PROFESSIONALS AND LAYPERSONS

While there is a tremendous need for more collaboration between professionals and self-help groups, a substantial foundation of interaction already exists. Two small studies, for instance, reported that about 50% of existing self-help groups were developed with some type of professional assistance (Madara, 1985; *Network,* 1983). A study of 43 groups revealed that social workers, clergy, teachers, physicians, registered nurses, and psychologists were involved with starting at least 10% of the existing groups in a three-county area of New York (Toseland & Hacker, 1982). Typically the professional who begins a self-help group does not share the physical or emotional condition of group members but rather has a professional interest in the group's focus (Toseland & Hacker, 1982).

In addition to developing self-help groups, professionals engage in a wide variety of supportive activities, including client referral, securing agency space, obtaining material support, consultation, accessing information, and linking to service agencies and other support groups. Sometimes groups are professionalized to the extent that they develop formal associations with professional agencies (e.g., Mended Hearts, Reach to Recovery) or transform into health associations.

Despite the collaborative basis that already exists between professionals and self-help groups, additional action is strongly recommended throughout the literature. One major barrier to collaboration is professional ignorance about support groups. One study of hospital social workers, for instance, reported only 3% had received significant instruction about self-help groups in their graduate school curricula (Black & Drachman, 1985). A national study of practicing social workers revealed that 40% of professional social workers did not make a single referral to a self-help group, with 25% not even knowing of a group to make a referral to (Toseland, 1985). Overall, 80% of the social work respondents reported that self-help groups were underused by themselves and their peers (Toseland, 1985). A poll of self-help group leaders revealed that over half of them believed that community agencies should be referring more clients to them, and many stated that professionals lacked understanding or knowledge about self-help groups (Toseland & Hacker, 1982). Borkman's (1982) review of the literature revealed that "the gerontological field is largely unaware of mutual self-help approaches in health and human sciences."

Stereotypical beliefs appear to be part of the problem as well. Many professionals, for instance, believe that self-help groups are antiprofessional (Medvene, 1984). One study reported that 60% of professional respondents believed self-help groups discourage members from seeking additional aid when needed (Toseland, 1985). These beliefs clash with earlier reports that group members are at least as likely to seek professional assistance as nonmembers (Lieberman & Borman, 1979).

Another barrier to collaboration is the belief that professionals will attempt to dominate self-help groups or change their ideology or methods of operation. Individual attempts by professionals to co-opt groups (Borkman, 1982) or alter their focus (Toseland & Hacker, 1982) do exist. There are legitimate concerns about the capacity of professionals to share leadership or to treat members in a nonpatient manner (Reever & Thomas, 1985).

These concerns about professional co-optation, however, are overshadowed by professional ignorance as the major barrier to collaboration. A study of hospital social workers revealed, however, that when professional ignorance is overcome through information, more referrals to self-help groups and offers of consultation are initiated (Black & Drachman, 1985). Collaborative relationships can be enhanced by greater awareness of the differences between the self-help and professional approaches to assistance and how they can be activated in a complementary fashion. The self-help approach has been described by analysts as informal, subjective, whole person oriented, personal, experiential, multifaceted, ongoing, and altruistic. Professional assistance, on the other hand, is characterized as task oriented, time-limited, impersonal, objective, formal, and treatment specific. When these approaches are viewed as contradictory, it is not surprising that professionals will lament the need for more training behind—and more restraint in—the helping approaches of self-help group members (Medvene, 1984). Nor is it surprising that these self-help group leaders complain that professionals tend to control or change laypersons rather than collaborate with them (Toseland & Hacker, 1982).

The potential for a complementary approach, however, is quite promising. Lay leadership will never take the place of trained professionals. And professionals need not view people, especially the elderly, as dependent on professional help and incapable of mutual aid or self-help. This "New Ageism" attitude (Kalish, 1979) can reinforce helplessness among older persons and their caregivers and reduce their self-esteem and sense of autonomy.

Four factors that support a complementary approach are (1) the need for peer assistance in an era of limited fiscal resources for professional skills, (2) the potential for peer groups to discover new knowledge and bring it to the attention of professionals, (3) the ability to meet existing service gaps or to serve persons unable or unwilling to access professional assistance, and (4) the ability of professionals to improve the effectiveness of groups through peer training in facilitation skills, provision of current knowledge, and, perhaps, feedback through evaluation studies.

Research will be a key factor in promoting a collaborative relationship. Lieberman (1985) suggests, for example, that professional involvement in self-help groups can contribute to group knowledge and skills and, therefore, group vitality and durability. While this observation appears true, it remains largely an untested empirical question. Another unexamined line of research is the motivational factor of the professionals who are already involved with self-help groups. Why and how was the contact initiated, how were professional-peer differences resolved, and what types of rewards do these professionals seek and experience (Medvene, 1984)? In other words, what are the factors of personal history, training, or circumstance that contribute to professional responsiveness to self-help groups? Also, how can self-help groups be improved or hindered by professional collaboration? How do self-help groups avoid bureaucratization, professionalization, or other assaults on their integrity? Examination of such questions is likely to lead to an increasing number of collaborative relationships between professionals and peer-led self-help groups.

CONGREGATIONAL SUPPORT

The association of self-help groups (or mutual aid societies, as they were once called) and religious institutions dates back at least as far as the 1700s (Frazier & Lincoln, 1974). Among contemporary self-help groups as well, the association with churches and synagogues remains strong. The roots of Alcoholics Anonymous (AA), for instance, can be traced to the work of a Lutheran minister. Many of the religious elements incorporated in AA have been adopted by numerous other support groups. Compassionate Friends, with over 400 chapters in America for parents who have suffered the death of a child, was started by an Anglican minister in England. GROW, a self-help group to support former mental patients, was initiated by a Jesuit priest.

A prime reason for the close association between congregations and self-help groups is the common focus on the same range of painful life circumstances and transitions: chronic illness, terminal illness, death, bereavement, loss, guilt, and ethical obligations. In addition, clergy and other religious leaders have special access to people in need, as hospital chaplains, funeral officials, and bereavement counselors.

Since religious leaders are sanctioned by society as the prime legitimizers of bereavement (Lieberman, 1985), they can provide legitimacy to the development and maintenance of self-help groups. Moreover, churches and synagogues often provide these groups with free space, publicity, help with fund raising, office equipment for mailings, or supplies. Not surprisingly, therefore, a survey of almost 2,500 groups in New Jersey whose meeting places were known revealed that 44% met in churches or temples (Madara & Peterson, 1986). Another survey of groups in New York reported 40% met in churches (Toseland & Hacker, 1982).

The association of religious institutions and self-help groups is not without problems or challenges. Often clergy are unaware of community resources that can benefit self-help members (Eisler et al., 1985). Also clergy give so much of their emotional and physical energy to their congregation membership often they neglect the emotional support they could receive themselves through support groups with their peers.

Furthermore, clergy are quite limited in their capacity to deal with large numbers of congregation members (Madara & Peterson, 1986). While a few have the skills to promote self-help groups to reach out to more people in need, many more do not have this knowledge or experience. Finally, the separation of church affiliation and social service is not always clearly delineated. Some support groups like THEOS, whose 140 chapters nationwide reach out to middle-age and young widowed persons, require groups to have a chaplain and to meet in a church under church auspices. Most groups, however, start out serving the needs of congregational members and eventually serve the general community. Typically these groups do not require any type of affiliation with the host religious organization (Madara & Peterson, 1986).

The association of the religious institution and self-help groups is especially fortuitous for older persons and their caregivers. First, the elderly constitute the largest age group in organized religion (Riessman et al., 1984). Second, the issues of loss and coping, which constitute the major domain of self-help groups, characterize the vast majority of challenges faced by the elderly and their caregivers. As people grow older, they lose some abilities to function physically; they lose spouses and other loved ones; and they invariably cope with their own chronic illness or the frailty of spouses, siblings, other family members, and friends. The association between self-help groups and religious institutions remains strong, and the likelihood is that the partnership will continue to flourish in the future.

RESEARCH

Given the scope of the self-help movement, the amount of rigorous research (pretests and posttests with control or comparison groups) is astonishingly little. There are several possible reasons for this dearth of research effort. Perhaps the professionals who are sensitive enough to collaborate with group members do not want to jeopardize matters with intrusive research questions. Perhaps results must be long term, over a period of years, and some researchers are discouraged by the cost and time involved. Perhaps the effort appears to be too complex to accomplish. How can you separate the impact of a self-help group from all other sources of influence? How do you obtain control groups (and is random assignment ever appropriate)? Just what do you measure: attitude change, behavioral change, group processes? How do you measure it: observation, participant observation, interviews, questionnaires, informants?

Despite the research challenges there have been a growing number of controlled studies of self-help groups. Lieberman and Gourash (1979) compared older peers in health promotion groups (SAGE) with those in comparison groups and reported reduced psychiatric symptoms and increased self-esteem. The group's impact, however, did not extend to physical health changes, such as physician visits or medication use. A study of widows in a support group reported that adjustment to bereavement occurred more rapidly for them than for those in a control group (Vachon et al., 1980). Active members in the support group THEOS reduced depression, anxiety, somatic symptoms, and use of psychotropic medications, while increasing self-esteem, coping ability, and psychological well-being (Lieberman & Borman, 1979). Finally, members of Mended Hearts (heart surgery aftermath) and Compassionate Friends (parents whose children have died) improved significantly on mental health measurements in comparison to those in control groups (Lieberman & Borman, 1979).

The agenda of research issues *not yet* examined, however, is much more extensive. There are few studies, for example, on self-help group process, other than those of an anecdotal nature, that shed light on the basic mechanisms producing change in participants. Lieberman (1985) postulates three theories of self-help change due to interpersonal processes: (1) the impact of disclosure, which produces empathy and catharsis and leads to feelings of normalization; (2) the impact of indoctrination, or the results of positive persuasiveness combined with an attractive ideology; and (3) the impact of networking, or the benefits of various types of social supports and respite assistance.

Also there has been little examination of developmental issues in self-help groups (Silverman, 1978). Do persons about to join groups go through stages of readiness before making their decision? Once in a group, do most members stay a short time (less than a year)? Among those who stay a long time, how does their participation in the group change? In addition to individuals in groups undergoing changes over time, does the group itself go through phases that impact on personal development?

The cost-effectiveness of self-help groups is very much an unresolved issue as well. Lieberman and Borman (1981) reported that participation in self-help groups tends to increase the use of professional resources. Members may learn about new benefits, entitlements, and resources through other group members. Members may also advocate for more insurance coverage or professional attention. On the other hand, a substitution effect may be achieved through these groups. Instead of more expensive professional attention, peers can provide emotional support, ongoing monitoring, assistance with medication compliance, and other kinds of peer-mediated instruction. These services are essential components to the management of chronic diseases and may be provided by professionals or layperson (Riessman et al., 1984). Other areas that impact on cost containment are earlier discharge from hospitals due to strengthened support groups, deinstitutionalization of higher functioning nursing home residents who were originally placed there because of inadequate support networks in the community, and fewer work days lost among caregivers who find support or respite through self-help groups.

A very much needed area of examination is who should be recruited into these groups and what techniques are effective in recruitment. It appears that the almost 90% of the elderly population with at least one chronic illness and their caregivers are ideal candidates for self-help groups. However, who prefers age-segregated versus age-integrated activities? Are older persons more reluctant to disclose feelings in a group setting? Are older persons willing to travel for a group meeting? Do older persons prefer churches, senior centers, or other community sites? Do age cohorts differ in their interest for advocacy activities? Can men be recruited as easily as women (Riessman et al., 1984)?

Why are poor persons, young and old, underrepresented in self-help groups? Given their higher prevalence of health problems and lower access to professional resources, they also appear to be ideal candidates for self-help groups. Perhaps it is just a matter of transportation and child care that prevents greater use of these groups among poor persons. Neighborhood-based church groups may be a means of grappling with these issues. Perhaps publicity and promotion by professionals and formal service agencies do not filter into the urban poverty pockets where social and health needs are greatest. Again, activating community churches and hospitals may be an effective way to publicize groups. Another argument is that poor persons do not want to take the initiative to colead groups, do not believe they have the power to effect change. One way of dealing with this possible barrier is to encourage groups with diverse economic and ethnic representation and to have assertive group members serve as role models. Regardless of whether potential barriers to participation in self-help groups by the poor are easily surmountable or not, self-help groups do not appear to have made many overtures to poor persons so far. Whether self-help groups must remain a middle-class phenomenon is still an unexamined question.

Finally, do peer groups do harm as well as good? The issue of quality control may be a substantial barrier to the collaboration between professionals and peer groups. Professionals are reluctant to refer clients to a source of assistance that has not been examined for quality. The few studies conducted in this area report that instances of abuse or neglect in the self-help movement are "relatively trivial and infrequent" (Lieberman, 1985). Clearinghouses have the potential to examine whether referrals to groups produce client satisfaction (Madara, 1986).

In short, there are many unexamined areas for researchers to tackle. Also, triangulated research efforts (i.e., multiple and complementary research approaches) are needed to grapple with the complexity of human behavior in groups. Field observations, interviews, informants, surveys, and other methodologies can help shed light on the complex process of mutual assistance. Finally, given the need for triangulated methods and in the spirit of the peer-oriented self-help movement itself, group members could be encouraged to examine their own helping process as well. The New Jersey Clearinghouse, for instance, distributed mini-grants to self-help groups to fund their own research projects. These group members may provide additional insight that can help researchers determine what makes a group effective.

CURRICULUM DEVELOPMENT

There is a widespread call in the literature for curriculum development so that students and practitioners can become more knowledgeable about self-help groups (Madara & Neigher, 1986; President's Commission on Mental Health, 1978; Riessman et al., 1984; Toseland, 1985). At both the undergraduate and graduate level, educational programs in the social, behavioral, educational, and health science professional fields can help students identify, use, and strengthen self-help groups. Also, federal organizations such as the Administration on Aging as well as professional societies can provide conferences, workshops, and continuing educational opportunities to foster curriculum development in the self-help group arena.

A nationwide survey of social workers revealed that over 90% wanted more information about self-help groups (Toseland, 1985). This is in contrast to the study of hospital social workers that reported that only 3% had received significant coverage of the topic in their graduate curricula (Black & Drachman, 1985). Borkman (1982) reports a comparable ignorance among gerontological practitioners. Borman's (1983) study of 160 professionals in Evanston, Illinois, reports that 100% of the practitioners wanted more information about self-help groups with which they were unfamiliar. Thus, both the need for and interest in curriculum development appear to be documented.

CLEARINGHOUSE

Based on the services provided by the two most comprehensive clearinghouses in the nation (which are actually "centers" because of their wide scope of activities), we find that four basic activities need to be offered: referral, group formation, public education, and research.

Through toll-free telephone information and referral services, *referrals* to existing groups can be made. The New Jersey center, for example, provided 1,400 referrals to groups in its first year of operation alone, and over 13,000 in its first 4 years of operation. Additional responses to requests for information were provided as well. After 4 years of operation, the New Jersey center had 3,150 referral sources in its data base, plus an additional 300 national and demonstration groups located outside of the state.

The computerized referral system provides instant retrieval of data to callers statewide. The computer search is structured by 80 general problem areas along five levels of geographical location: local, county, state, regional, or national groups. In addition, the computer easily updates information as groups develop, change location, or terminate. Referrals are also enhanced through computer printouts of copy-ready directories. The New Jersey center distributed 3,000 directories in its first 3 years of operation.

Group formation can be stimulated through conferences, workshops, educational forums, and speaker's bureaus in the community. Group formation can also occur through computer-aided networking. The computer first identifies subject areas in which callers are requesting groups but no existing groups have been formed. Next the callers are linked and provided with information and technical assistance. This assistance may include identifying free church or agency space; locating available clerical or mailing services; providing the capacity to piggyback an answering service onto existing help lines; and identifying professionals, members of other self-help groups, or national organizations willing to contribute information and resources to start groups.

Another group formation service available by computer is telecommunications, since an increasing number of households include a personal computer. Thus, persons who are disabled, have transportation problems, or are afflicted with rare conditions that have potential members dispersed over a wide geographical area are now able to link by computer.

Clearinghouses can provide *community education* in a wide variety of ways. The New Jersey center, for instance, organized 20 state and regional conferences during its first 3 years of operation and reached out to 2,000 participants. In addition, the center provided 80 seminars and workshops, which were attended by 3,000 people. They organized a speaker's bureau, distributed directories free of charge as a means of public education, and distributed newsletters and other educational materials.

A wide variety of how-to materials is also being developed and disseminated by self-help clearinghouses. Topics include how to start a group, overcoming transportation barriers, maintaining records, fund raising for special projects, facilitating the group process, developing shared leadership capacity, and printing community resource guides. The Illinois Self Help Center has a library with a comprehensive resource collection on mutual help groups. The collection includes reports, government documents, journals, magazine articles, books, and films.

The Illinois center also implements professional training and retraining to promote better collaboration between professionals and self-help groups. The

New Jersey center experimented with a 24-hour computer-accessible bulletin board to publicize existing groups and to promote various services. There is great potential for other types of innovative community educational projects through self-help clearinghouses.

Another service of a self-help clearinghouse or center is *research.* In addition to encouraging research in the broader scientific community and performing research with internal professional staff, the computerized clearinghouse provides a rich resource of data for future studies. Comprehensive data files can include information on the types and frequency of phone calls from laypersons and from professionals, the types and frequency of problems being presented, the types and frequency of referrals being made, and the satisfaction level of consumers toward their self-help referrals.

9

CONCLUSION

The basic premise of this book is that we are entering the era of low technology, low-cost, community-based long-term health care. This era has been heralded by two well-documented trends: (1) *The staggering and sustained growth of health care expenditures.* The startling rise in health care expenditures was nowhere more apparent than in the hospital and nursing home sectors. Thus, high-cost, institutional-based care became a major factor in precipitating the health care cost containment era of the 1980s. (2) *The need to provide population-relevant health care to an aging America.* The impact of the demographic mandate on the health care cost containment era has been well documented also. Demographic analysis of the "aging of the aged" clearly reveals the challenge of mounting health care costs associated with the fastest growing segment of the population—persons age 80 and over—who demand the most intensive and extensive long-term care services.

The rising health costs and the growing demand for long-term health care are especially challenging in an era of sluggish economic growth and limited resources. This combination of fiscal, demographical, and economical turbulence could last a half century, until the early 2040s, when the last of the baby boomers (those born between 1946 and 1964) join the tail end of the gerontology boom.

Beleaguered service providers and deficit conscious policymakers will have a simple choice to make, and perhaps the approach will be more semantic than substantive. The positive choice is to develop new techniques, different emphases, and a renewed spirit to meet the unrelenting demand for community-based long-term care services. The negative approach is to focus on rationing, or who does not get what. The latter approach must come to terms with the question: Does the public have the right to heroic medical care, unlimited access to expanding technological options, and utilization of an increasing percentage of the federal and state dollar on health care?

The sluggish American economy has been complicated by startling increases in the defense budget throughout the first half of the 1980s, questionable tax cuts, and a staggering federal budget deficit. No matter what the final outcome of the Gramm-Rudman-Hollings Deficit Reduction Act or similar legislation, certain unpleasant realities will emerge. Taxes will unquestionably be raised; domestic programs deserving expansion will be hard pressed merely to maintain current expenditure levels; and cost containment will have to be tolerated, whether embraced by the majority or not.

An economic crisis is not merely a problem, though, but also an opportunity to develop innovative programs. First, aging Americans need new programs that are *holistic and interdisciplinary,* more so than younger adults, who enter the health care system with specific health problems. Second, aging Americans want *educational programs that help them remain in their homes*—the most comfortable, private, and personal environment available to them. Education is equally important for older spouses and siblings, as well as younger adult children, who need caregiver training, support, and respite. Third, education and support must be ongoing and accessible—two qualities that characterize the burgeoning *self-help group movement.*

Fourth, education is also important for professionals who are not trained in geriatrics or who need training and information to *promote health, prevent disease, or enhance self-care capabilities.* These professionals must join the aging population and their family members in learning new skills and knowledge in the areas of exercise, stress management, nutrition, and self-care. Health promotion requires new collaborative relationships among health professionals, between professionals and laypersons, and among family members.

Fifth, the era of government limits means new initiatives must come from the *corporate sector* and from *congregations* of all faiths. The corporate sector is motivated by economic concerns—rising medical expenditures for an aging work force and an increasing number of retirees. The incentive for congregations is provided by their emphasis on the family and their capacity and desire to reach those unable or unwilling to be served by formal service agencies.

The low-technology, low-cost, community-based long-term health care era is not an era of government abandonment. There will always be a need for *government leadership.* Leaving families and communities to their own devices is just as likely to undermine individual autonomy and self-respect as an overreliance on big government and its past proclivity for medical and institutional solutions to health problems. Families and volunteers cannot take on the whole burden of the health care transformation. They need access to government services.

Moreover, there will always be a need for national leadership in the areas of education, training, research, and policy. In the policymaking arena it is inconceivable that a nation would settle for a hodgepodge of conflicting laws and practices in areas that reflect fundamental values and issues of morality and ethics. Health care treatment in the last 6 months of life, for instance, needs national direction. The policy of providing unlimited, high-tech, crisis-oriented medical care to terminally ill patients versus one that emphasizes the hospice approach—informal supports, primary care, and mental health promotion—should not be decided idiosyncratically within insulated communities.

Our current health care cost containment policies present policymakers with either a dilemma or an opportunity, depending on whether they view the proverbial half a glass of water as being half empty or half full. The pessimistic policymaker, for instance, sees the huge unsatisfied thirst for home- and community-based long-term care support and ponders the dilemma: How can we meet even the smallest fraction of a pent-up demand for chronic care services in the community when we are having trouble limiting public expenditures for sophisticated acute care and institutional long-term care? The optimistic (and opportunistic) policymaker, on the other hand, views the public's growing awareness of the fiscal limits in health care as an opportunity to help individuals, families, and neighborhoods develop innovative solutions to new problems.

It is my contention that informal caregiving, self-help groups, congregations and corporations, health promotion, and education will be the vital components of the long-term care system that emerges in the era of cost containment.

BIBLIOGRAPHY

Abramowitz, M. (1986, November 18). In an effort to cut costs, the insurance industry is in flux. *Washington Post,* p. 16.

ACTION. (1984). *Descriptive evaluation of RSVP and FGP volunteers working with Headstart.* Washington, DC: Office of Policy and Planning Evaluation Division.

ACTION. (1985). *Senior companion program impact evaluation.* Alexandria, VA: SRA Technologies.

Aday, L., et al. (1980). *Health care in the U.S.: Equitable for whom?* Beverly Hills: Sage.

Ahart, G. (1981, December 29). *How health maintenance organizations control costs* (Report to R. Schweiker, secretary of HHS). Washington, DC: U.S. General Accounting Office.

Altman, D. (1983). Health care for the poor. *Annals, 468,* 103–121.

American Association of Retired Persons. (1988). *Understanding senior housing,* Washington, DC: Consumer Affairs/Program Department.

Amster, L., & Krauss, H. (1974). The relationship between life crises and mental deterioration in old age. *International Journal of Aging and Human Development, 5,* 51–55.

Arling, G., & McAuley, W. (1983). The feasibility of public payments for family caregiving. *Gerontologist, 23,* 300–306.

Atchley, R. (1985). *Social forces and aging* (4th ed.). Belmont, CA: Wadsworth.

Avorn, J., & Langer, E. (1982). Increased disability in nursing home patients: A controlled trial. *Journal of the American Geriatrics Society, 30,* 397–400.

Banta, D., et al. (1983). Policy applications of the diffusion and control of medical technology. *Annals, 468,* 165–181.

Barbaro, E., & Noyes, L. (1984). A wellness program for a life care community. *Gerontologist, 24,* 568–571.

Bausell, R. (1986). Health seeking behavior among the elderly. *Gerontologist, 26,* 556–559.

Beck, N. (1986, April 16). *IBM health care strategy.* Paper presented at the meeting of the Council on Wage and Price Stability, Washington, D.C.

Bengtson, V. (1979). Ethnicity and aging: Problems and issues in current social science inquiry. In D. Gelfand & A. Kutzik (Eds.), *Ethnicity and aging* (pp. 9–31). New York: Springer.

Bennett, R., et al. (1986). *Program of continuing education in geriatric medicine and long term care services: A series of interdisciplinary seminars, designed to update community physicians' knowledge of geriatric medicine with a view to use of non-medical services and resources available in the community* (Final Report). Washington, DC: Administration on Aging, Office of Human Development Services.

Benson, H. (1976). *The relaxation response.* New York: Avon.

Berki, S. (1983) Health care policy in American. *Annals, 468.*

Besdine, R. (1987). Challenges in health care of the elderly: Educational responsibilities and opportunities. In *Workshop for key staff of geriatric education centers* (pp. 26–30). Educational Development Center: Boston.

Black, R., & Drachman, D. (1985, Spring). Hospital social workers and self-help groups. *Health and Social Work,* pp. 95–103.

Blumenfield S., et al. (1982). The geriatric team in the acute care hospital: An educational and consultation modality. *Journal of the American Geriatrics Society, 30*(10), 660–664.

Blumenthal, H. (1965). The shape of the gerontological society. *Gerontologist, 5,* 3, 48.

Borkman, T. (1982). Where are older persons in mutual self-help groups. In A. Kolker & P. Ahmed (Eds.), *Aging.* New York: Elsevier.

Borman, L. (1983). *Study of 160 professionals in Evanston, Illinois.* Unpublished manuscript, Self-Help Center, 1600 Dodge Avenue, Suite S-122, Evanston, IL 60201.

Brody, E. (1981). Women in the middle and family help to older people. *Gerontologist, 21,* 471–480.

Brody, E. (1985). Parent care as a normative family stress. *Gerontologist, 25,* 19–29.

Brody, E., et al. (1983). Women's changing roles and help to elderly parents: Attitudes of 3 generations of women. *Journal of Gerontology, 38,* 597–607.

Brody, E., & Schoonover, C. (1986). Patterns of parent care when adult daughters work and when they do not. *Gerontologist, 26,* 372–381.

Brody, E., et al. (1978). The family care unit: A major consideration in the long-term care support system. *Gerontologist, 18,* 556–561.

Brown, L. (1983). Competition and health care policy—experience and expectations. *Annals,* 468, 48–59.

Buccola, A., & Stone, J. (1975). Effect of jogging and cycling programs on physiological and personality variables in aged men. *Research Quarterly, 46,* 134–139.

Business and health year end update, quality of care. (1985). *Business and Health, 3*(2), 35.

Butler, R. (1975). *Why survive? Being old in America.* New York: Harper & Row.

Butler, R., et al. (1979). Self-care, self-help, and the elderly. *International Journal of Aging and Human Development, 10,* 95–117.

Butler, R. M., & Lewis, M. (1982). *Aging and mental health.* St. Louis: Mosby.

Butterfield-Picard, H., & Magno, J. (1982). Hospice the adjective, not the noun: The future of a national priority. *American Psychologist, 37*(11), 1254–1259.

Califano, J., Jr. (1986). *America's health care revolution: Who lives? Who dies? Who pays?* New York: Random House.

Callahan, J., et al. (1980). Responsibility of families for their severely disabled elders. *Health Care Financing Review, 1,* 29–48.

Cantor, M. (1979a). Neighbors and friends: An overlooked resource in the informal support system. *Research on Aging, 1,* 434–463.

Cantor, M. (1979b). The informal support system of New York's inner city elderly: Is ethnicity a factor? In D. Gelfand & A. Kutzik (Eds.), *Ethnicity and aging* (pp. 153–174). New York: Springer.

Cantor, M. (1981). *Factors associated with strain among family, friends and neighbors caring for the frail elderly.* Paper presented at the 34th Annual Meeting of the Gerontological Society of America, Toronto.

Cantor, M. (1983). Strain among caregivers: A study of experience in the United States. *Gerontologist, 23,* 597–604.

Cantor, M., & Mayer, M. (1978). Factors in differential utilization of services by urban elderly. *Journal of Gerontological Social Work, 1*(1), 47–62.

Capitman, J. (1986). Community-based long-term care models, target groups, and impacts on service use. *Gerontologist, 26,* 389–397.

Capitman, J., et al. (1986). Case management approaches in coordinated community-oriented long-term care. *Gerontologist, 26,* 398–404.

Carp, F. (1976). Housing and living environments of older people. In R. Binstock & E. Shanas (Eds.), *Handbook of aging and the social sciences.* New York: Van Nostrand.

Chambre, S. (1984). Is volunteering a substitute for role loss in old age? An empirical test of activity theory. *Gerontologist, 24,* 292–298.

Chappell, N. (1985). Social support and the receipt of home care services. *Gerontologist, 25*(1), 47–54.

Checkbook. (1980). (Newsletter published by Washington Center for the Study of Services). *3* (1).

Christensen, A., & Rankin, D. (1979). *Easy does it yoga for older people.* New York: Harper & Row.

Cicirelli, V. (1983). A comparison of helping behavior to elderly parents of adult children with intact and disrupted marriages. *Gerontologist, 23,* 619–625.

Clark, N., & Rakowski, W. (1983). Family caregivers of older adults: Improving helping skills. *Gerontologist, 23,* 637–642.

Coe, R., et al. (1984). Complimentary and compensatory functions in social network relationships among the elderly. *Gerontologist, 24,* 396–400.

Cohen, C., et al. (1985). Social networks and adaptation. *Gerontologist, 25,* 297–304.

Cole, T. (1983). The "enlightened" view of aging: Victorian morality in a new key. *Hastings Center Report, 13,* 34–40.

Collins, H., & Pancoast, D. L. (1976). *Natural helping networks: A strategy for prevention.* Washington, DC: National Association of Social Workers.

Congressional Budget Office. (1979). *PSRO.* Washington, DC: U.S. Government Printing Office.

Cook, K., et al. (1983). A theory of organizational response to regulation: The case of hospitals. *Academy of Management Review, 8*(2), 193–205.

Cooper, K. H. (1976). *The new aerobics.* New York: Bantam.

Coward, R. (1983). Cautions about the role of natural helping networks in programs for the rural elderly. In N. Stinnett et al. (Eds.), *Family strengths: Positive support systems* (pp. 291–306). Lincoln: University of Nebraska.

Creedon, M., (1987). *Issues for an aging America: Employees and eldercare.* Bridgeport, CT: University of Bridgeport, Center for the Study of Aging.

Dancy, J., Jr. (1977). *The black elderly.* Ann Arbor: University of Michigan-Wayne State University, Institute of Gerontology.

Davis, K., & Rowland, D. (1986). *Medicare policy: New directions for health and long term care.* Baltimore: Johns Hopkins.

D.C. Office on Aging. (1978). *Needs assessment for older persons* (Title III, AOA, Older Americans Act funded project). Washington, DC: Author.

Department of Mental Health (1979). *Statistical tabulations from a survey of California adults on their own mental health and well-being.* Sacramento: Author.

deVries, H. A. (1970). Physiological effects of an exercise training regimen upon men aged 52 to 88. *Journal of Gerontology, 25,* 325–336.

Dichter, E., et al. (1981). *Helping the informal support network: A new approach to serving the elderly* (Vol. 1). New York: Community Research Applications.

Dimatteo, M., & Hayes, R. (1981). Social support and serious illness. In B. H. Gottlieb (Ed.), *Social networks and social support.* Beverly Hills: Sage.

Doka, K. (1985–1986). The church and the elderly: The impact of changing age strata on congregations. *International Journal of Aging and Human Development, 22*(4), 291–300.

Doty, P., et al. (1984). An overview of long-term care. *Health Care Financing Review, 6,* 69–78.

Duke University. (1978). *The OARS methodology: Multidimensional functional assessment* (2nd ed.). Durham: Center for the Study of Aging and Human Development

Dunham, A., & Morone, J. (1983, January). *DRG evolution: Political evaluation.* Unpublished manuscript, Health Research and Education Trust of New Jersey.

Dychtwald, K. (1986). *Wellness and health promotion for the elderly.* Rockville, MD: Aspen.

Ehrlich, P. (1983). Elderly health advocacy group: An integrative planning model of elderly consumers and service delivers. *Gerontologist, 23,* 569–572.

Eisler, T., et al. (1985). Training clergy to help the elderly and their families. *Journal of Applied Gerontology, 4*(2), 58–62.

Enthoven, A. (1980). *Health plan: The only practical solution to the soaring cost of medical care.* Reading, MA: Addison-Wesley.

Erikson, M. (1987). Workplace health promotion. In P. Lazes et al. (Eds.), *The handbook of health education* (pp. 281–310). Rockville, MD: Aspen.

Ettinger, K., et al. (1981). The development of teaching programs in geriatric dentistry in the United States from 1974 to 1979. *Special Care in Dentistry, 1*(5), 221–224.

Eustis, N., et al. (1984). *Long-term care for older persons: A policy perspective.* Monterey, CA: Brooks/Cole.

Evans, E. (1979). *The Family Circle guide to self-help.* New York: Ballantine Books.

Fallcreek, S., & Mettler, M. (1982). *A healthy old age* (a sourcebook for health promotion with older adults). Seattle Center for Social Welfare Research, School of Social Work, University of Washington.

Fallcreek, S., & Stam, S. (Eds.). (1982). *The Wallingford Wellness Project* (an innovative health promotion program with older adults). Seattle: Center for Social Welfare Research, School of Social Work, University of Washington.

Feder, J., & Scanlon, W. (1980). Regulating the bed supply in nursing homes. *Milbank Memorial Fund Quarterly Health and Society, 58*(1), 54–88.

Feder, J., et al. (1982). *Health in the Reagan experiment: An examination of economic and social policies.* Washington, DC: Urban Institute.

Fielding, E. (1982). Effectiveness of employee health improvement programs. *Journal of Occupational Medicine, 5,* 237–265.

Fields, C. (1987). *Interfaith caregiving dissemination project.* DHHS, AOA model project, 1986–1988). Washington, DC: University of the District of Columbia.

Fitting, M., et al. (1986). Caregivers for dementia patients: A comparison of husbands and wives. *Gerontologist, 26,* 248–252.

Fox, P., et al. (1984). *Health care cost management: Private sector initiatives.* Ann Arbor: Health Administration Press.

Frazier, E., & Lincoln, C. (1974). *The Negro church in America/The black church since Frazier.* New York: Schocken Books.

Friedman, D. (1986). Eldercare: The employee benefit of the 1990's. *Across the Board, 23*(6), 44–51.

Fries, F., & Crapo, M. (1986). The elimination of premature disease. In K. Dychtwald (Ed.), *Wellness and health promotion for the elderly* (pp. 19–37). Rockville, MD: Aspen.

Fullerton, H., & Tschetter, J. (1983, November). The 1995 labor force: A second look. *Monthly Labor Review,* pp. 3–10.

Gadow, S. (1983) Frailty and strength: The dialectic in aging. *Gerontologist, 23,* 144–147.

Gallup. (1977). *Survey of public awareness.* Princeton: Author.

Gilligan, C. (1982). *In a different voice.* Cambridge: Harvard University.

Ginsburg, E. (1983). Urban health care: Change and more change. In A. Greer & S. Greer (Eds.), *Cities and sickness: Health care in urban America.* Beverly Hills: Sage

Goldbeck, W. (1984). Health Care Coalitions. In P. Fox et al. (Eds.), *Health care cost management: Private sector initiatives.* Ann Arbor: Health Administration Press.

Goodman, C. (1984). Natural helping among other adults. *Gerontologist, 24* 138–143.

Gurewitsch, E. (1983, July/August). Geriatric day care: The options reconsidered. *Aging,* pp. 21–26.

Gutkin, C. (1987). *Volunteer caregivers in housing for the elderly* (DHHS, AOA model project, 1986–1987). Boston: Hebrew Rehabilitation Center for the Aged.

Gwyther, L., & George, L., (1986). Symposium introduction: Caregivers for dementia patients: Complex determinants of well-being and burden. *Gerontologist, 26,* 245–247.

Haber, D. (1979, November/December). Old age in China. *Aging,* pp. 7–9.

Haber, D. (1983a). *Church-based program for caregivers of the elderly* (AOA model project, Final Report). Washington, DC: University of the District of Columbia.

Haber, D. (1983b). Promoting mutual help groups among older persons. *Gerontologist, 23,* 251–253.

Haber, D. (1983c). Yoga as a preventive health care program. *International Journal of Aging and Human Development, 17*(4), 169–176.

Haber, D. (1984a). Church-based programs for caregivers of non-institutionalized elders. *Journal of Gerontological Social Work, 7*(4), 43–55.

Haber, D. (1984b). Church based mutual help groups for caregivers of non-institutionalized elders. *Journal of Religion and Aging, 1*(1), 63–70.

Haber, D. (1985). *Allocating resources for the aged: Strategies for state leaders*. Washington, DC: National Association of State Units on Aging.

Haber, D. (1986a). Health promotion to reduce blood pressure level among older blacks. *Gerontologist, 26,* 118–121.

Haber, D. (1986b). In-home and community-based long-term care services: A review of recent AOA projects involving self-determination. *Journal of Applied Gerontology, 5*(1), 37–50.

Haber, D. (1986c). The integration of a field experience in nursing homes. *Journal of Long Term Care Administration, 14*(2), 23–25.

Haber, D. (1988a). The interfaith volunteer caregiver program. *Journal of Religion and Aging, 3*(3–4), 151–156.

Haber, D. (1988b). A health promotion program in ten nursing homes. *Activities, Adaptation and Aging, 2*(1), 73–82.

Haber, D., & Wicht, J. (1987). Worksite wellness and aging. *Wellness Perspectives, 4*(4), 31–34.

Hagan, R. (1984, September 21). *Hearing statement* (U.S. Senate Special Committee on Aging). Washington, DC: U.S. Government Printing Office.

Hanson, S., et al. (1983). Racial and cohort variations in filial responsibility norms. *Gerontologist, 23,* 626–631.

Haugk, K. (1976). Unique contributions of churches and clergy to community mental health. *Community Mental Health Journal, 12*(1).

Hawkins, B., & Jacobson, S. (1980). *The role of caregivers in the black community* (Final Report, AOA Grant No. 90-A-1375). Washington, DC.

Hays, J. (1984, April). Aging and family resources: Availability and proximity of kin. *Gerontologist, 24,* 149–153.

Health Advocate. (1983–1984). (Newsletter of the National Health Law Program). *139,* pp. 7–10.

Healthworks, health promotion programs in small business. (1984). Seattle: Puget Sound Health Systems Agency.

Healthy people: The surgeon general's report on health promotion and disease prevention. (1979). (Public Health Service No. 79-55071). Washington, DC: Health Education and Welfare.

Heaney, R., et al. (1977). Calcium balance and calcium requirements in middle-aged women. *American Journal of Clinical Nutrition, 30,* 1603–1611.

Helphano, M., & Porter, C. (1981). The family group within the nursing home: Maintaining family ties of long-term care residents. *Journal of Gerontological Social Work, 4,* 51–62.

Hereford, R. (1982). *Competition: A new approach to controlling health care costs.* Washington, DC: National Conference of State Legislatures, George Washington University.

Hess, R. (1982). Self-help as a service delivery strategy. *Prevention in Human Services, 1,* 1–2.

Hodgson, J. L., & Buskirk, E. R. (1977). Physical fitness and age, with emphasis on cardiovascular function in the elderly. *Journal of the American Geriatrics Society, 25,* 385–392.

Hofer, A. (1980, November). *The family support system: Comparative analysis of research projects funded by the Administration on Aging.* Paper presented to the U.S. Senate Special Committee on Aging.

Hofer, A. (1982, November). *Strengthening the self capacity of the family caretaker of elderly living at home.* Paper presented at the meeting of the Gerontological Society of America, Boston.

Holmes, T., & Masuda, M. (1973). Life change and illness susceptibility. In B. Dohrenwend & B. Dohrenwend (Eds.), *Stressful life events: Their nature and effects.* New York: Wiley.

Hooyman, N. (1980). Mutual help organizations for rural older woman. *Educational Gerontology, 5,* 429–447.

Hooyman, N., & Lustbader, W. (1986). *Taking care: Supporting older people and their families.* New York: Free Press.

Hornbrook, M. (1983). Allocative medicine: Efficiency, disease severity and the payment mechanism. *Annals, 468,* 12–29.

Horowitz, A. (1985). Sons and daughters as caregivers to older parents: Differences in role performance and consequences. *Gerontologist, 25,* 612–617.

Horowitz, A., & Dobrof, R. (1982). *Role of family caregivers in providing long term care to the frail and chronically ill elderly living in the community* (Final Report, HCFA Grant No., 18-97541). Baltimore.

Horowitz, A., et al. (1983, November). *Employment and daughter caregivers: A working partnership for older people?* Paper presented at the 36th annual meeting of the Gerontological Society of America, San Francisco.

Hospice benefits. (1985). *Business and Health, 3*(2), 34.

International Society of Certified Employe Benefit Specialists. (1985, November). *Results: Census of certified employee benefit specialists.*

IVCP in perspective. (1986). *Interfaith Volunteer Caregivers Program Bulletin, 3*(1), 3. Benedictine Hospital, P.O. Box 1939, Kingston, NY 12401.

Izzo, J. L. (1982). Hypertension in the elderly: A pathophysiologic approach to therapy. *Journal of the American Geriatric Society, 30,* 352–359.

Jackson, J. (1980). *Minorities and aging.* Belmont, CA: Wadsworth.

Jacobs, B. (1985). *The national potential of home equity conversion* (Report prepared for the U.S. Senate Special Committee on Aging and the U.S. House Select Committee on Aging). Rochester, NY: University of Rochester.

Jacobson, E. (1938). *Progressive relaxation.* Chicago: University of Chicago.

Jacobson, E. (1972). *You must relax.* New York: McGraw-Hill.

Jajich, C. L., et al. (1984). Smoking and coronary heart disease mortality in the elderly. *Journal of the American Medical Association, 252*(20), 2831–2834.

Jarrett, W. (1985). Caregiving within kinship systems: Is affection really necessary? *Gerontologist, 25,* 5–10.

Johnson, C., & Catalano, D. (1983). A longitudinal study of family supports to impaired elderly. *Gerontologist, 23,* 612–618.

Juster, R., & Lanning, J. (1982, August). *Health care cost containment strategies: A bibliography.* Chicago: Council of Planning Librarians.

Kalish, R. (1979). The new ageism and the failure models: A polemic. *Gerontologist, 19,* 175–202.

Kane, R., et al. (1979). *The PSRO and the nursing home.* Unpublished manuscript, Rand Corporation, Santa Monica.

Kane, R., et al. (1983). Predicting the outcomes of nursing-home patients. *Gerontologist, 23,* 200–206.

Kane-Williams, E., et al. (1986). *Staying healthy after fifty.* Washington, DC: American Association of Retired Persons.

Kappelman, M. M., et al. (1981). A non-traditional geriatric teaching model: Interpersonal service/education sites. *Journal of Medical Education, 56,* 467–477.

Kemper, D. (1984). *An evaluation of the growing younger health promotion program for older adults.* Executive summary. Boise: Healthwise.

Kemper, D. (1986). The healthwise program: Growing younger. In K. Dychtwald (Ed.), *Wellness and health promotion for the elderly* (pp. 263–274). Rockville, MD: Aspen.

Kemper, D. (1987). A evaluation of the growing wiser mental wellness program for older adults. Unpublished manuscript, P.O. Box 1989, Boise, ID 83701.

Kemper, D., et al. (1986). *Growing wiser: The older persons guide to mental wellness.* Boise: Healthwise.

Kemper, D., et al. (1987). *Growing younger handbook* (3rd ed.). Boise: Healthwise.

Kemper, P., et al. (1987). Community care demonstrations: What have we learned? *Health Care Financing Review, 8*(4), 87–100.

Kendig, H., & Rowland, D. (1983). Family support of the Australian aged: A comparison with the United States. *Gerontologist, 23,* 643–649.

Kiefhaber, A. K., & Goldbeck, B. (1986). *Work site wellness in health care cost management: Private sector initiatives.* Washington, DC: Health Administration Press.

Kim, P. (1980). Toward rural gerontological education: rationale and model. *Educational Gerontology, 5,* 387–397.

Kizer, W. (1987). *The healthy workplace.* New York: John Wiley and Sons.

Knight, B., & Walker, D. (1985). Toward a definition of alternatives to institutionalization for the frail elderly. *Gerontologist, 25,* 358–363.

Knowles, L. (1982). Gerontological nursing. *International Journal of Nursing Studies, 20*(1), 45–54.

Kristen, M. (1980, January). *How much can business expect to earn from smoking cessation?* Paper presented at the National Interagency Council on Smoking and Health's Workshop, Smoking and the Workplace, Chicago.

Krolner, B., et al. (1983). Physical exercise as prophylaxis against involutional bone loss: A controlled trial. *Clinical Science, 64,* 541–546.

Krout, J. (1985). Relationships between informal and formal organizational networks. In W. Sauer & R. Coward (Eds.). *Social support networks and the care of the elderly* (pp. 178–196). New York: Springer.

Kuhn, T. (1970). *The structure of scientific revolutions* (2nd ed.). Chicago: University of Chicago.

Lang, A., & Brody, E. (1983). Characteristics of middle-aged daughters and help to their elderly mothers. *Journal of Marriage and the Family, 45,* 193–202.

Langer, E., & Rodin, J. (1976). The effects of choice and enhanced personal responsibility for the aged: A field experiment in an institutional setting. *Journal of Personality and Social Psychology, 34,* 191–198.

Laurie, W. (1978). Employing the Duke OARS methodology in cost comparisons: Homeservices and institutionalizations. *Advances in Research, 2,* 2.

Lederman, S., et al. (1983). *Generations, 1*(3), 48–49.

Lederman, S., & Farrar, M. (1985). *The wisdom project of the American Red Cross in greater New York: A blue print for a community-based health care and health education program.* Unpublished manuscript.

Leutz, W., et al. (1985). *Changing health care for an aging society.* Lexington, MA: Lexington Books.

Levin, L. (1986). Reproduced in J. Simmons et al. The Dartmouth self-care for senior citizens program. In K. Dychtwald (Ed.), *Wellness and health promotion for the elderly.* Rockville, MD (p. 235). Rockville, MD: Aspen.

Levin, R. (1987). *Wellness Programs for older workers and retirees.* Washington, DC: Washington Business Group on Health.

Lieberman, M. (1985). Self-help groups: An overview, *Generations, 10*(1), 45–49.

Lieberman, M., & Borman, L. (Eds.). (1979). *Self-help groups for coping with crisis.* San Francisco: Jossey-Bass.

Lieberman, M., & Borman, L. (1981). The impact of self-help groups on widow's mental health. *National Research and Information Center's National Reporter, 4,* 7.

Lieberman, M., & Gourash, N. (1979). Effects of change groups on the elderly. In M. Lieberman & L. Borman (Eds.), *Self-help groups for coping with crisis* (pp. 387–405). San Francisco: Jossey-Bass.

Litwak, E. (1965). Extended kin relations in an industrial democratic society. In E. Shanas & G. Streib (Eds.), *Social structure and the family: Generational relations.* Englewood Cliffs, NJ: Prentice Hall.

Litwak, E., & Figueria, J. (1968). Technological innovation and theoretical functions of primary groups and bureaucratic structures. *American Journal of Sociology, 4,* 468–481.

Lowenstein, F. W. (1982). Nutritional status of the elderly in the United States of America. *Journal of the American College of Nutrition, 1,* 165–177.

Lowenthal, M., et al. (1975). *Four stages of life: A comparative study of women and men facing transitions.* San Francisco: Jossey-Bass.

Lubitz, J., & Prihoda, R. (1984). The use and cost of Medicare services in the last two years of life. *Health Financing Review, 3,* 117–131.

Luft, H. (1985). HMOs: Friends or foes? *Business and Health, 3*(2), 5–10.

Lupu, D. (1984–1985). *Hospice services for patients without family caregivers* (AOA and DHHS Grant Project 90-AM-0060). Chevy Chase, MD: Montgomery Hospice Society.

Mace, N., & Rabins, P. (1984, December). *A survey of day care for the demented adult in the United States.* Washington, DC: National Council on the Aging.

Macken, C. (1982). *Long term care survey.* Washington, DC: Health Care Financing Administration.

Madara, E. (1985). The self-help clearinghouse operation: Tapping the resource development potential of I & R services. *Journal of the Alliance of Information and Referral Systems, 1,* 42–58.

Madara, E. (1986). A comprehensive systems approach to promoting mutual aid self-help groups: The New Jersey self-help clearinghouse model. *Journal of Voluntary Action Research, 15*(2), 57–63.

Madara, E., & Neigher, N. (1986). Hospitals and self-help groups: Opportunity and challenge. *Health Progress, 67*(3), 42–45.

Madara, E., & Peterson, B. (1986). *Clergy and self-help groups: Practical and promising relationships.* Unpublished manuscript, Denville, NJ.

Manheim, L. (1982, April). *Reimbursement incentives in the financing of long term care.* Unpublished manuscript, Northwestern University, Center for Health Services and Policy, Evanston, IL.

Mathematical Policy Research. (1986). *The evaluation of the national long term care demonstration: final report* (DHHS Contract No. 100-80-0157). Plainsboro, NJ.

McAuley, W., & Arling, G. Use of in-home care by very old people. *Journal of Health and Social Behavior, 25,* 54–64.

McAuley, W., & Blieszner, R. (1985, April). Selection of long-term care arrangements by older community residents. *Gerontologist, 25,* 188–193.

McCarthy, H. (1980). *Coping with stroke: Effects of self-help group participation among disabled seniors.* Paper presented at the 33rd Annual Scientific Meeting of the Gerontological Society of America, San Diego.

McClure, W. (1983). The competition strategy for medical care. *Annals of the American Academy of Political and Social Sciences, 468,* 30–47.

McNerney, W. (1983, March 14). *A two tier system of health care: Are we headed toward one system for the privileged and another for the underprivileged?* Evanston, IL: Northwestern University, Center for Health Services and Policy Research.

Medvene, L. (1984, Spring). Self-help and professional collaboration. *Social Policy,* pp. 15–18.

Mellinger, G., & Balter, M. (1983). *Collaborative project* (GMIRSB Report). Washington, DC: National Institute of Mental Health.

Miller, D. (1981). The sandwich generation: Adult children of the aging. *Social Work, 15*(3), 419–423.

Mindel, C. (1979). Multigenerational family households: Recent trends and implications for the future. *Gerontologist, 19,* 456–463.

Mindel, C. (1980). Extended familism among urban Mexican Americans, Anglos and blacks. *Hispanic Journal of Behavioral Sciences, 2,* 21–34.

Mindel, C., et al. (1986). Informal and formal health and social support systems of black and white elderly: A comparative cost approach. *Gerontologist, 26,* 279–285.

Minkler, M. (1983). Health promotion and elders: A critique. *Generations, 3*(3), 13–15, 67.

Mitchell, J., & Register, J. (1984). An exploration of family interaction with the elderly by race, SES, and religion. *Gerontologist, 24,* 48–54.

Moberg, D. (1983, Fall). The ecological fallacy: Concerns for program planners. *Generations, 8*(1), 12–14.

Molinari, V., et al. (1983). Geropsychiatry training of medical students in a community mental health center setting. *Gerontology and Geriatric Education, 3,* 291–295.

Montgomery, R., & Prothero, J. (1985). *Developing respite services.* Unpublished manuscript, Pacific Northwest Long Term Care Center, Seattle.

Mor, V. (1986, August). A national study of residential care for the aged. *Gerontologist, 26,* 405–417.

Morgan, J., et al. (1979). *Results from two national surveys of philanthropic activity.* Ann Arbor: Survey Research Center, University of Michigan.

Moss, M., et al. (1985). The quality of relationships between elderly persons and their out-of-town children. *Gerontologist, 25*(2), 134–140.

Myers, E. (1983). Gerontological counseling training: The state of the art. *Personnel and Guidance Journal, 61*(7), 398–401.

Myers, J., & Blake, R. (1986). Counselor preparation: preparing counselors for work with older people. *Counselor Education and Supervision, 26*(2), 137–144.

Nahemow, L., & Mintz, J. (1981). *People care for people: Providing a missing link in the chain of natural support systems.* New York: New York Office of Health Affairs, Division of Gerontology, New York University Medical Center.

Naisbett, J. (1982). *Megatrends.* New York: Warner Books.

National Center for Health Statistics. (1986, September 19). *Advance data from vital and health statistics* (Report No. 126). Hyattsville, MD: Public Health Service, National Heart Lung and Blood Institute Demonstration Projects in Workplace High Blood Pressure Control. (For further information contact Judith H. LaRosa, NHLBI, Building 31, Room, 4A18, Bethesda, MD 20205.)

National Conference of State Legislators. (1984, January). *Major health issues for the states: 1984, health care cost containment project.* Unpublished manuscript, Denver.

National Council on the Aging. (1982, March–April). *Public policy agenda, 1986–87. Perspective on aging.* Washington, DC: Author.

National Governor's Association. (1984, February). *Governor's guide to health care cost containment strategies.* Unpublished manuscript, Washington, DC.

National Heart, Lung, and Blood Institute. (1981). *Exercise and Your Heart* (NIH Publication No. 81-1677). Washington, DC: National Institutes of Health.

National Heart, Lung, and Blood Institute. (1983). *Work place high blood pressure control.* Washington, DC: National Center for Health Statistics.

National Institute on Aging. (1984, February). *Report on education and training in geriatrics and gerontology.* Washington, DC: Author.

National Institute on Aging. (1987, September). *Personnel for health needs of the elderly through the year 2020, executive summary report.* Washington, DC: Department of Health and Human Services, Public Health Service.

National long-term care channeling demonstration. Preliminary analysis. (1986, January 30). (Report to assistant secretary for planning and evaluation). Washington, DC: Department of Health and Human Services.

National Retired Teachers Association/American Association of Retired Persons. (1981). *National survey of older Americans.* Washington, DC: Author.

Natural supports program. (1981). Unpublished manuscript, AOA Model Project, Community Service Society, New York.

Nelson, G. (1982, March). Support for the aged: Public and private responsibility. *Social Work,* pp. 137–142.

Nelson, E., et al. (1986). *Medical and health guide for people over fifty.* Glenview, IL: Scott, Foresman.

Nestle, M. (1983). Dietary recommendations for older Americans. *Generations, 3*(3), 20–22.

Network. (1983, Spring). (Newsletter of the New Jersey Self-Help Clearinghouse), *3,* 2.

New rules of exercise. (1986, August 11). *U.S. News and World Report,* pp. 52–56.

Newcomer, R., et al. (1983). *Policy Development in the Medicare, Medicaid and Social Security Programs* (Policy paper No. 6). San Francisco: University of California, Aging Health Policy Center.

Newquist, D. (1985). *Health and extended worklife.* An informational paper prepared for use by the U.S. Senate Special Committee on Aging. Washington, DC: U.S. Government Printing Office.

Nichols, E. (1981). Multidisciplinary professional education in gerontology. *Gerontology and Geriatric Education, 2,* 87–92.

Nocks, B. (1986, April). The effects of a community-based long term care project on nursing home utilization. *Gerontologist, 26,* 150–157.

O'Brien, J., & Wagner, D. (1980). Helpseeking by the frail elderly: Problems in network analysis. *Gerontologist, 20,* 78–83.

O'Bryant, S. (1985). Neighbors' support of older widows who live alone in their homes. *Gerontologist, 25,* 305–310.

Ochsner, M. (1983, October). *Financing health care for the aged.* New York: Columbia University, Brookdale Institute on Aging and Adult Development.

Office of Human Development Services. (1984, May). *Federal support for self-help under the coordinated discretionary program of OHDS.* Unpublished manuscript, Office of Human Development Services, Office of Program Development, Washington, DC.

Office of Human Development Services. (1987, December). Coordinated discretionary funds program: Availability of funds and requests for applications fiscal year 1987. *Federal Register.*

Office of State Health Planning, State-Wide Health Coordinating Council. (1982, May). *Health plan for Massachusetts.* Unpublished manuscript, Boston, p. 8.

Oktay, J., & Volland. (1981, July). *The community care program: Foster homes as an alternative to institutional care.* Paper presented at the 12th Annual International Congress of Gerontology, Hamburg, West Germany.

Older Adults Service and Information System. (1986). *Disseminating the OASIS program for older adults.* (AOA Final Report Grant No. 90AM 008201). Washington, DC: Author.

Older Women's League. (1985, June). *Fact sheet.* Washington, DC: Author.

Oriol, W. (1985). *The complex cube of long term care.* Washington, DC: American Health Planning Association.

Ozawa, M. (1985). *Case management services by the volunteer elderly* (AOA, DHDS, DHHS grant project). St. Louis: Washington University.

Palmore, E. (1980). The social factors in aging. In E. Busse & D. Blazer (Eds.), *Handbook of geriatric psychiatry* (pp. 222–248). New York: Van Nostrand Reinhold.

Payne, B. (1986, November). *Consortia models for teaching, research and field experience in seminaries.* Paper presented at the Annual Meeting of the Gerontological Society of America, Chicago.

Pearson, R. (1982). Support: Exploration of a basic concept in counseling and informal help. *Personnel and Guidance Journal, 61,* 83–86.

Pegels, C. (1980). *Health care and the elderly.* Rockville, MD: Aspen Systems.

Pfeiffer, E., et al. (1985, August). *Respite care.* Tampa: University of South Florida, Suncoast Gerontology Center.

Pierce, B., & Hekman, E. (1983, December). *Health cost containment legislation: 1983 legislative update, 50 states.* Denver: National Conference of State Legislatures.

Pilisuk, M., & Froland, C. (1978). Kinship social networks, social support and health. *Social Issues and Medicine, 12b,* 273–280.

Pilisuk, M., & Minkler, M. (1980). Supportive networks: Life ties for the elderly. *Journal of Social Issues, 36,* 95–116.

Polich, C., et al. (1987). *Who will pay? The employers' role in financing health care for the elderly.* Minneapolis: Interstudy Center for Aging and Long-Term Care.

Polich, C., & Iverson, L. (1987). *The provision of long-term care in risk based HMO's.* Minneapolis: Interstudy Center for Aging and Long-Term Care.

President's Commission on Mental Health. (1978). *Commission report* (Vol. 1, p. 144). Washington, DC: U.S. Government Printing Office.

Preston, D., & Mansfield, P. (1984). An exploration of stressful life events, illness and coping among the rural elderly. *Gerontologist, 24,* 490–494.

Prisuta, R. (1984, October). *Evaluation of the AARP widowed persons services.* Washington DC: American Association of Retired Persons, Research and Data Department.

Puska, P., et al. (1983). Controlled, randomized trial of the effect of dietary fat on blood pressure. *Lancet i*(8312/5), 1–5.

Pynoos, J., et al. (1984). Intergenerational neighborhood networks: A basis for aiding the frail elderly. *Gerontologist, 24,* 233–237.

Pynoos, J. (1987). *Telephone networks for caregivers, Administration on Aging project.* Washington, DC: Office of Human Development Services.

Quinn, J. (1985, February 4). Medicare HMOs can provide quality health care at lower costs. *Washington Post,* Washington business section, p. 59.

Rabin, D. L., & Stockman, P. (1987). *Long term care of the elderly: A fact book.* New York: Oxford.

Raschko, R. (1985). Systems integration at the program level: Aging and mental health. *Gerontologist, 25,* 460–463.

Rathbone-McCuan, E., et al. (1985). Social support for the frail elderly. In W. Sauer & R. Coward (Eds.), *Social support networks and the care of the elderly.* New York: Springer.

Reever, K., & Thomas, E. (1985). Training facilitators of self-help groups for caregivers to elders. *Generations, 10*(1), 50–52.

Reichstein, K., & Bergofsky, L. (1983). Domiciliary care facilities for adults: An analysis of state regulations. *Research on Aging, 5,* 25–43.

Retsinas, J., & Garrity, P. (1986). Going home: Analysis of nursing home discharges. *Gerontologist, 26,* 431–436.

Rich, F. (1985a, April 29). Chrysler saves $58 million in battle against health care waste. *Washington Post,* Washington business section, p. 3.

Rich, F. (1985b, July 27). Nursing home expenses deplete elderly's funds. *Washington Post,* Washington business section, p. 10.

Rich, F. (1985c, July 27). Gap in long term care for elderly reported in study. *Washington Post,* Washington business section, p. 11.

Riessman, F., et al. (1984, Spring). Self-help and the elderly. *Social Policy,* pp. 19–26.

Riessman, F., & Moody, H. (1982). *Self-help and the elderly: Considerations for practice and policy.* Washington, DC: National Council on the Aging.

Robinson, B., & Thurnher, J. (1979). Taking care of aged parents: A family cycle transition. *Gerontologist, 19*(1), 586–593.

Rodin, J., & Langer, E. (1977). Long-term effects of a control-relevant intervention among the institutionalized aged. *Journal of Personality and Social Psychology, 35,* 897–902.

Ronan, L. (1982, July). *State health care cost containment: A review of strategies.* Unpublished manuscript, Institute for Health Planning, Madison.

Rosen, I. (1974). Some contributions of religion to mental and physical health. *Journal of Religion and Health, 13*(4), 289–294.

Rosenthal, C. (1986). Family supports in later life: Does ethnicity make a difference? *Gerontologist, 26* 19–24.

Rosow, I. (1967). *Social integration of the aged.* New York: Free Press.

Rouse, I. L., et al. (1983). Blood-pressure-lowering effect of a vegetarian diet: Controlled trial in normotensive subjects. *Lancet i*(8314/5), 5–10.

Rubenstein, D. (1971). An examination of social participation of black and white elderly. *Aging and Human Development, 2,* 172–188.

Rubin, A., & Shuttlesworth, G. (1983). Engaging families as support resources in nursing home care: Ambiguity in the subdivision of tasks. *Gerontologist, 23,* 632–636.

Ruskin, P. (1983, November 25). Aging and caring. *Journal of the American Medical Association, 25,* 2440.

Satin, D. G. (1986, February). *The difficulties of interdisciplinary education: Lessons from three failures and a success.* Paper presented at the 12th Annual Meeting of the Association for Gerontology in Higher Education, Atlanta.

Satin, D. G., et al. (1985, February). *Teaching an interdisciplinary approach to geriatrics: A solution to Babel.* Paper presented at the 12th Annual Meeting of the Association for Gerontology in Higher Education, Washington, DC.

Sauer, W., & Seelbach, W. (1983, December). Racial and cohort variations in filial responsibility norms. *Gerontologist, 23,* 621–631.

Saxon, S., & Etten, M. (1987). *Physical change and aging: A guide for the helping professions* (2nd ed.). New York: Tiresias Press.

Schoen, E., et al. (1983, June). *Cost containment project report,* Office of Medical Assistance, Pennsylvania Department of Public Welfare.

Scholl, N. (1980). Smoking habits in the glosterub population of men and women, born in 1914. *Acta Medical Scandinavica, 208,* 254–256.

Scott, D. M., et al. (1983). The development and evaluation of an interdisciplinary health training program: A pharmacy perspective. *American Journal of Pharmaceutical Education, 47,* 42–48.

Scott, J., & Roberto, K. (1985). Use of informal and formal support networks by rural elderly poor. *Gerontologist, 25,* 624–630.

Segal, S. (1986, February). Retirement programs in the '80s. *Personnel Administration.*

Selye, H. (1976). *The stress of life* (rev. ed.). New York: McGraw-Hill.

Shanas, E. (1979). Social myth as hypothesis: The case of the family relations of older people. *Gerontologist, 19,* 169–174.

Shanas, E. (1980). Older people and their families: The new pioneers. *Journal of Marriage and the Family, 43,* 9–15.

Shanas, E., & Sussman, M. (1977). *Family, bureaucracy, and the elderly.* Durham: Duke University.

Sheehan, N. (1986). Informal support among the elderly in public senior housing. *Gerontologist, 26,* 171–175.

Shepard, K., et al. (1985). Successful components of interdisciplinary education. *Journal of Allied Health, 14*(3), 297–302.

Shriner, D. M., et al. (1983). Promoting faculty support and participation in geriatric teaching programs. *Gerontology and Geriatrics Education, 4,* 51–57.

Sidney, K. H., Shephard, R. J., & Harrison, J. E. (1977). Endurance training and body composition of the elderly. *American Journal of Clinical Nutrition, 30,* 326–333.

Silverman, A., et al. (1981). *As parents grow older: A manual for program replication.* Ann Arbor: University of Michigan, Institutes of Gerontology.

Silverman, P. (1978). *Mutual help groups: A guide for mental health workers* (DHEW Publication No. ADM-78-646). Rockville, MD: National Institute of Mental Health.

Simmons, J., et al. (1983). Self care: Tools, strategies and methods. *Generations, 3*(3), 46–47, 64.

Simmons, J., et al. (1986). The Dartmouth self-care for senior citizens program: Tools, strategies and methods. In K. Dychtwald (Ed.), *Wellness and health promotion for the elderly,* pp. 235–246. Rockville, MD: Aspen.

Simonson, W. & Pratt, C. (1982). Geriatric pharmacy curriculum in U.S. pharmacy schools: A nationwide survey. *American Journal of Pharmaceutical Education, 46,* 249.

Simson, A., & Wilson, B. (1983, February). *Report on education and training in geriatrics.* Unpublished administrative document, National Institute on Aging.

Slivinske, L., & Kosberg, J. (1984). Assessing the effect of a personal health management system within retirement communities: A preliminary investigation. *Gerontologist, 24,* 280–285.

Sloan, F. (1983). Rate regulation as a strategy for hospital cost control: Evidence from the last decade. *Milbank Memorial Fund Quarterly, 61*(2), 195–221.

Smith, E. (1982). Exercise for prevention of osteoporosis: A review. *Physician and Sports Medicine, 10,* 72–83.

Smits, H. (1981). The PSRO in perspective. *New England Journal of Medicine, 305,* 253–259.

Soldo, B., & Myllyluoma, J. (1983). Caregivers who live with dependent elderly. *Gerontologist, 23,* 605–611.

Spence, D. L., et al. (1986). *Multidisciplinary health seminars for the elderly.* (Final report to the Rhode Island Foundation). Providence: University of Rhode Island, Program in Gerontology.

Steiger, N., & Lipson, J. (1985). *Self-care nursing: Theory and practice.* Bowie, MD: Brady Communications.

Stephens, M., & Bernstein, M. (1984). Social support and well-being among residents of planned housing. *Gerontologist, 24,* 144–148.

Stone, R., et al. (1986). *Caregivers of the frail elderly: A national profile.* Paper presented at the American Society on Aging, San Francisco.

Sussman, M. (1976). The family life of old people. In R. Binstock & E. Shanas (Eds.), *Handbook of aging and the social sciences* (pp. 218–243). New York: Van Nostrand Reinhold.

Taylor, M. (1986). Contradictions in federal policies put elderly in risk of health care neglect. *Home Health Care Services Quarterly, 7*(2), 5–12.

Taylor, R. (1985). The extended family as a source of support to elderly blacks. *Gerontologist, 25,* 488–495.

Thoits, P. (1982). Conceptual, methodological, and theoretical problems in studying social support as a buffer against life stress. *Journal of Health and Social Behavior, 23,* 145–149.

Thomas, A. M., & Ship, I. I. (1981). Current status of geriatric education in American dental schools. *Journal Dental Education, 45*(9), 589–591.

Thornberry, O., et al. (1986, May 14). Health promotion and disease prevention, provisional data from the National Health Interview Survey: United States, January–June, 1985. National Center for Health Statistics, U.S. Department of Health and Human Services, Public Health Service. *Advance Data, 119.*

Tierney, J., et al. (1982). Certificate of need—no panacea but not without merit. *Journal of Public Health Policy, 15,* 178–181.

Tobin, S. (1982, July–August). Churches and agencies often at odds in aiding the elderly. *Aging,* pp. 46–47.

Tobin, S., et al. (1986). *Enabling the elderly: Religious institutions within the community service system.* Albany: State University Press of New York.

Tobin, S., & Ellor, J. (1983). The church and the aging network: More interaction needed. *Generations, 8*(1), 26–27.

Toffler, A. (1980). *The third wave.* New York: William Morrow.

Toseland, R. (1985, November). *Professional social workers and self-help groups.* Paper presented at the annual meeting of the Gerontological Society of America, New York.

Toseland, R., & Hacker, L. (1982, July). Self-help groups and professional involvement. *Social Work,* pp. 341–347.

Treants, S., et al. (1981). Physical manifestations of aging: Preparation for practice through a team-taught course with a cross-professional field component. *Gerontology and Geriatric Education, 2,* 99–101.

Turner, N. (1985). Wellness: The revolution of the 80's. *ICAD Ideas, 5*(1), 1–4.

Tynan, E., et al. (1981, March). *Nursing home reimbursement.* Hyattsville, MD: National Center for Health Services.

Tyson, K., & Merrill, J. (1983). *Health care institutions: Survival in a changing environment.* Unpublished manuscript, Washington, DC, Center for Health Policy Studies, Georgetown University.

U.S. Bureau of Labor Statistics. (1984, January). *Employment and earnings* (Table 3). Washington, DC: Author.

U.S. Comptroller General. (1981). *HSA impact on cost containment* (Report No. HRD-81-55). Washington, DC: U.S. General Accounting Office.

U.S. General Accounting Office. (1981, December 29). *How health maintenance organizations control costs* (Report No. HRD-82-31). Washington, DC: Author.

U.S. General Accounting Office. (1982, September 24) *A primer on competitive strategies for containing health care costs* (Report No. GAO/HRO-82-92). Washington, DC: Author.

U.S. Senate Special Committee on Aging. (1985). *Developments in aging: 1984.* Washington, DC: U.S. Government Printing Office.

U.S. Senate Special Committee on Aging. (1986). *Developments in aging: 1985.* Washington, DC: U.S. Government Printing Office.

Vachon, M., et al. (1980, November). A controlled study of self-help intervention for widows. *American Journal of Psychiatry, 137*(11), 1179-1184.

Waldo, D., & Lazenby, H. (1984). 1984 demographic characteristics and health care use and expenditures by the aged in the U.S.: 1977-1984. *Health Care Financing Review, 6*(1), 1-30.

Wallace, R. (1970). *The physiological effects of transcendental meditation.* Unpublished doctoral dissertation, University of California, Los Angeles.

Warner-Reitz, A. (1981). *Healthy lifestyle for seniors: An interdisciplinary approach to healthy aging.* New York: Meals for Millions/Freedom from Hunger Foundation.

Watson, J. (1968). *Double helix: A personal account of discovery of the structure of DNA.* New York: Atheneum.

Wechsler, R., & Minkler, M. (1986). A community-oriented approach to health promotion: The Tenderloin senior outreach project, pp. 301-312. In K. Dychtwald (Ed.), *Wellness and health promotion for the elderly.* Rockville, MD: Aspen.

Weeks, J., & Cueller, J. (1981). Minority differences in caregiving: The role of family members in the helping networks of older people. *Gerontologist, 21,* 388-394.

Weihl, H. (1983). Three issues from the Israeli scene. *Gerontologist, 23,* 576-579.

Weiler, P. (1983). Education and training in wellness for elders. *Generations, 8*(3), 34-36.

Weinrobe, M. (1984). Home equity conversion. In D. Feinstein et al. (Eds.), *Long term care financing and delivery systems.* Washington, DC: Health Care Financing Administration.

Weis, W. L. (1981, May). Can you afford to hire smokers? *Personnel Administrator.*

Weissert, W. (1985). Seven reasons why it is so difficult to make community based long-term care cost-effective. *Journal of Health Services Research, 20,* 4.

Widowed Persons Service. (1984-1985). *AARP directory of services for the widowed in the U.S. and Canada.* Washington, DC: American Association of Retired Persons.

Wiener, J., et al. (1987). Private long term care insurance: Cost, coverage, and restrictions. *The Gerontologist, 27*(4), 487-493.

Williamson, J., & Danaher, K. (1978). *Self-care in health.* London: Croomhelm.

Winsburg, G. (1985). The hidden costs of HMOs. *Business and Health, 3*(2), 18–21.

Wood, L. (1980). *Lifestyle management strategies at New York Telephone.* Paper presented at the Leadership Strategies Health Conference, Millwood, VA.

Young, C. (1986). Organizational volunteers for the rural, frail elderly: Outreach, case finding and service delivery. *Gerontologist, 26,* 342–344.

Zimmer, A., & Sainer, J. (1978, November). *Strengthening the family as an informal support for their aged.* Paper presented at the 31st Annual Meeting of the Gerontological Society, Dallas.

Zischka, P., & Jones, I. (1984). Volunteer community representatives as ombudsman for the elderly in long-term care facilities. *Gerontologist, 27,* 9–12.

APPENDIXES

A

ERA OF COST CONTAINMENT: RESOURCES

NATIONAL ASSOCIATIONS CONCERNED WITH AGING

Administration on Aging
330 Independence Avenue, SW
Washington, DC 20201
(202) 245-0724

Acts as advocate for the elderly; serves as the principal agency for implementing programs of the Older Americans Act.

Alzheimer's Disease and Related Disorders Association, Inc.
70 East Lake Street
Chicago, IL 60601
(312) 853-3060

Promotes research education and advocacy; develops family support for relatives of victims.

American Association for Geriatric Psychiatry
P.O. Box 376A
Greenbelt, MD 20770
(301) 220-0952

An association of psychiatrists who specialize in treating mental disorders of older patients.

American Association of Homes for the Aging
1050 17th Street, NW
Suite 770
Washington, DC 20036
(202) 296-5960

An association of 3,200 nonprofit nursing homes, independent housing facilities, continuing care facilities, congregate housing, skilled nursing, and related services.

American Association of Retired Persons
1909 K Street, NW
Washington, DC 20049
(202) 728-4300

Membership organization of persons age 50 and over. Publishes materials for older persons and caregivers; offers discounted health insurance, hotel rates, car rentals; implements service programs.

American Geriatrics Society
770 Lexington Avenue
Suite 400
New York, NY 10021
(212) 308-1414

A society of health care professionals, over 95% physicians, devoted to the clinical care of the elderly. American Geriatrics Society has formed a section for teachers of geriatric medicine and a section for long-term care physicians.

American Health Care Association
1200 15th Street, NW
Washington, DC 20005
(202) 833-2050

A nonprofit federation of 50 state associations plus Washington, D.C., serving nearly 9,500 licensed nursing homes and allied facilities.

American Society for Geriatric Dentistry
211 East Chicago Avenue
Chicago, IL 60611
(312) 353-6547

Focuses on education of dental professionals to meet the needs of the elderly patient.

American Society on Aging
833 Market Street
Suite 512
San Francisco, CA 94103
(415) 543-2617

A national, nonprofit membership organization of practitioners, educators, researchers, and others in the field of aging. National and regional conferences attract practitioners and others.

Asociacion Nacional por Personas Mayores
(National Association for Hispanic Elderly)
2727 W. 6th Street
Suite 270
Los Angeles, CA 90057
(213) 487-1922

Provides information, resource guides, bibliographies, and advocacy for Hispanic and other low-income persons age 55 and over.

Association for Gerontology in Higher Education
600 Maryland Avenue, SW
West Wing
Washington, DC 20024
(202) 484-7505

Membership organization of over 200 colleges and universities. Its purpose is to increase the commitment of higher education in the field of aging through education, research, and public service. The association conducts an annual conference, updates its *National Directory of Educational Programs in Gerontology,* and publishes a newsletter.

Center for Health Promotion and Education
Building 14
Center for Disease Control
Atlanta, GA 30333

Provides a list of health education contacts in each state.

Concern for Dying
250 W. 57th Street
Suite 831
New York, NY 10107
(212) 246-6973

Society for the Right to Die
250 W. 57th Street
Suite 323
New York, NY 10107
(212) 246-6973

Concern for Dying and the Society for the Right to Die are organizations providing information about living wills and death with dignity.

Concerned Relatives of Nursing Home Patients
P.O. Box 18820
Cleveland Heights, OH 44118
(216) 321-0403

Monitors quality of care in nursing homes; an advocate for patients' rights in 28 states.

Gerontological Society of America
1275 K Street, NW
Suite 350
Washington, DC 20005-4006
(202) 842-1275

A 6,000-member multidisciplinary organization devoted to aging, research, and education. Annual conference attracts academic researchers, practitioners, and others.

Gray Panthers
311 South Juniper
Suite 601
Philadelphia, PA 19107
(215) 545-6555

Gray Panthers
806 15th Street, NW
Suite 430
Washington, DC 20005
(202) 783-6226

Coalition of young and old persons working together to combat ageism. Newsletter and other publications available.

House Select Committee on Aging
300 New Jersey Avenue, SE
Room 712, Annex 1
Washington, DC 20515
(202) 226-3375

Publishes reports and conducts hearings on legislative developments, health care, and other issues.

National Association of Area Agencies on Aging
600 Maryland Avenue, SW
Suite 208
Washington, DC 20024
(202) 484-7520
Promotes communication among 660 area agencies on aging through conferences and publications; engages in research. Area agencies on aging are responsible for planning, implementing, and coordinating service delivery systems to meet the needs of older persons. To locate your local AAA, look in the telephone listing for your city or county under Department or Office on Aging, Social Services, or similar titles.

National Association for Home Care
519 C Street, NE
Stanton Park
Washington, DC 20002
(202) 547-7424
Provides for homemaker, home health, and hospice services; lists home health care organizations.

National Association of Meal Programs
204 E Street, NE
Washington, DC 20002
(202) 547-6157
Provides technical assistance, information, and legislative leadership in the area of home- and community-based meal programs for older persons.

National Association of Medical Equipment Supplies
618 S. Alfred Street
Alexandria, VA 22314
(703) 736-6263
Provides advocacy for home health care industry; focuses on supplies of durable medical equipment.

National Association of State Units on Aging
2033 K Street, NW
Suite 304
Washington, DC 20006
(202) 785-0707

Promotes communication among 57 state and territorial departments on aging through educational forums, training programs, and research projects.

National Caucus and Center on Black Aged
1424 K Street, NW
Suite 500
Washington, DC 20005
(202) 637-8400

Provides information, advocacy, employment programs, and related services for blacks and low-income elders.

National Council of Senior Citizens
925 15th Street, NW
Washington, DC 20005
(202) 347-8800

Offers information on Medicare, Social Security, and nursing homes; advocacy for older persons.

National Council on the Aging
600 Maryland Avenue, SW
West Wing 100
Washington, DC 20024
(202) 479-1200

Provides numerous publications on such topics as caregiving, adult day care, and health promotion; holds an annual conference for practioners and laypersons; sponsors National Institute on Adult Day Care and National Center for Health Promotion and Aging.

National Foundation for Long Term Health Care
1200 15th Street, NW
Washington, DC 20005
(202) 833-2050

A nonprofit organization that develops programs in research and education in long-term health care.

National Hearing Aid Society
20361 Middlebelt
Livonia, MI 48152
(800) 521-5247
(313) 478-2610

Offers consumer information and advocacy; has a data resource center and toll free hearing aid helpline. A certifying body for audiologists.

National Home Caring Council
235 Park Avenue, South
New York, NY 10003
(212) 674-4990

Membership organization of home care agencies, other interested organizations, and individuals. Helps locate local home care agencies and publishes related materials.

National Hospice Organization
1901 North Fort Myer Drive
Suite 307
Arlington, VA 22209
(703) 243-5900

Serves as an information source on local hospices; monitors legislation; issues publications.

National Indian Council on Aging
P.O. Box 2088
Albuquerque, NM 87103
(505) 242-9505

Provides information on American Indian and Alaskan aged.

National Institute of Mental Health
Mental Disorders of the Aging Research Branch
Room 11C-03
5600 Fishers Lane
Rockville, MD 20857
(301) 443-1185

Supports a complete range of treatment settings that serve mental disorders of the aging.

National Institute on Aging
Building 31, Room 5C35
Bethesda, MD 20205
(301) 496-1752

Conducts and supports research on aging. Brochures, fact sheets (Age Pages), conferences, and other forms of community education are promoted.

National Pacific/Asian Resource Center on Aging
1341 G Street, NW
Washington, DC 20005
(202) 393-7838

Focuses on health and social services for Pacific/Asian elders.

Office of Disease Prevention and Health Promotion
Department of Health and Human Services
300 7th Street, SW
Washington, DC 20201
(202) 245-7611

Provides health promotion program materials and information about state and local level health initiatives with older people. Each state has a designated contact person to disseminate information and coordinate health programs.

Older Women's League
730 11th Street, NW
Suite 300
Washington, DC 20001
(202) 783-6686

Offers policy papers and consumer publications on midlife and older women's health issues, caregiving, and death and dying; primary focus is on education and advocacy.

Senate Special Committee on Aging
SD-G37 Dirksen Senate Office Building
Washington, DC 20510
(202) 224-5364

Conducts studies on the problems and opportunities of older people. Publishes *Developments in Aging*, an annual report on the latest data about aging and public policy.

Subcommittee on Health and Long Term Care
715 House Office Building
Annex 1
Washington, DC 20515
(202) 226-3381

Conducts continuing studies of matters pertaining to problems of older persons.

U.S. Health Care Financing Administration
200 Independence Avenue, SW
Hubert Humphrey Building, Room 314G
Washington, DC 20201
(202) 245-6726

Office of Beneficiary Services
6325 Security Boulevard
Baltimore, MD 21207

The Health Care Financing Administration oversees the Medicare and Medicaid programs and publishes free pamphlets.

U.S. Veterans Administration
810 Vermont Avenue, NW
Washington, DC 20420
(202) 393-4130

Administers the laws that authorize benefits for former members of the Armed Forces and their dependents.

Villers Foundation
1334 G Street, NW
Washington, DC 20005
(202) 737-6340

Focuses on political advocacy and empowerment among elders. Spearheads a coalition of national aging organizations (Advocates Senior Alert Process) to provide advocates with timely special reports on key issues, advocacy tips, and action alerts that require immediate response to legislators and other policymakers.

PEER REVIEW ORGANIZATIONS (PROs)*

PROs seek to ensure that Medicare patients receive necessary and good quality medical care, as well as adequate hospital discharge planning. If you are unable to reach a state organization regarding a patient complaint on the quality of Medicare services, contact the Office of Medical Review Health Standards and Quality Bureau, Meadows East Building, 6325 Security Boulevard, Baltimore, MD 21207; (303) 966-6851.

Alabama

Alabama Quality Assurance Foundation
236 Goodwin Crest Drive
Suite 300
Twin Towers East
Birmingham, AL 35209
(205) 942-0785

Alaska

Professional Review Organization for Washington
2150 N. 107th Street
Suite 200
Seattle, WA 98133
(206) 364-9700

Arizona

Health Services Advisory Group, Inc.
1020 E. Missouri
P.O. Box 16731
Phoenix, AR 85014
(602) 279-1615

Arkansas

Arkansas Foundation for Medical Care, Inc.
101 N. 6th Street
P.O. Box 1508
Fort Smith, AR 72902
(501) 785-2471

California

California Medical Review, Inc.
1388 Sutter Street
Suite 1100
San Francisco, CA 94109
(415) 923-2000

Colorado

Colorado Foundation for Medical Care
6825 East Tennessee Avenue
Building 2, Suite 400
Denver, CO 80224
(303) 321-8642

Connecticut

Connecticut Peer Review Organization
384 Pratt Street
Meriden, CT 06450
(203) 237-2773

Delaware

Delaware Review Organization
Independence Mall
Suite 92-100
1601 Concord Pike
Wilmington, DE 19803
(302) 654-4488

District of Columbia

Delmarva Foundation for Medical Care
108 North Harrison Street
Easton, MD 21601
(301) 822-7223

Florida

Professional Foundation for Health Care
2907 Bay to Bay Boulevard
Tampa, FL 33629
(813) 831-6273

Georgia

Georgia Medical Care Foundation/PRO
4 Executive Park Drive, NE
Suite 1300
Atlanta, GA 30329
(404) 982-6500

Hawaii

Health Services Advisory Group, Inc.
1020 E. Missouri
P.O. Box 16731
Phoenix, AZ 85014
(602) 279-1615

Idaho

(Fiscal Intermediary)
Idaho Medicare Peer Review Organization
P.O. Box 7777
Boise, ID 83707
(208) 345-6727

Illinois

Crescent Counties Foundation for Medical Care
350 Shuman Boulevard
Suite 240
Naperville, IL 60540
(312) 357-8770

Indiana

Indiana PRO
11550 North Meridian Street
Tower 1
Carmel, IN 46032
(317) 844-4777

Iowa

Iowa Foundation for Medical Care
3737 Woodland Avenue
Suite 500
West Des Moines, IA 50265
(515) 233-2900

Kansas

Kansas Foundation for Medical Care
2953 S.W. Wanamaker Drive
Topeka, KS 66614
(913) 273-2552

Kentucky

Kentucky Peer Review Organization
10101 Linn Station Road
Louisville, KY 40223
(502) 426-4888

Louisiana

Louisiana Medical Review Foundation
733 East Airport Avenue
Suite 202
Baton Rouge, LA 70806
(504) 923-2078

Maine

Health Care Review, Inc.
The Weld Building
345 Blackstone Boulevard
Providence, RI 02906
(401) 331-6661

Maryland

Maryland Health Care Foundation
40 West Chesapeake Avenue
Suite 608
Towson, MD 21204
(301) 583-7273

Massachusetts

Physician Peer Review
1340 Centre Street
Newton Centre, MA 02159
(617) 965-5000

Michigan

Michigan Peer Review Organization
40500 Ann Arbor Road
Suite 200

Plymouth, MI 48170
(313) 459-0900

Minnesota

Foundation for Health Care Evaluation
2221 University Avenue, SE
Suite 300
Minneapolis, MN 55414
(612) 379-4443

Mississippi

Mississippi Foundation for Medical Care, Inc.
P.O. Box 4665
Jackson, MS 39216
(1900 North West Street, Zip 39202)
(601) 948-8894

Missouri

Missouri Patient Care Review Foundation
1026C Northwest Drive
Jefferson City, MO 65101
(314) 634-4411

Montana

Montana-Wyoming FMC
P.O. Box 5117
Placer Center
21 N. Main Street
Helena, MT 59604
(406) 443-4020

Nebraska

Nebraska FMC, Inc.
1221 N Street
Suite 801, CTU Building
Lincoln, NE 68501
(402) 474-7471

Nevada

Nevada Physicians Review Organization
3660 Baker Lane
Reno, NV 89509
(702) 826-1996

New Hampshire

New Hampshire Foundation for Medical Care
672 Central Avenue
P.O. Box 578
Dover, NH 03820
(603) 749-1641

New Jersey

Peer Review Organization of New Jersey
The Jefferson Building East
330 Milltown Road
East Brunswick, NJ 08816
(201) 238-5570

New Mexico

New Mexico Medical Review Association
2350 Alamo, SE
Albuquerque, NM 87106
(505) 842-6236

New York

Empire State Medical, Scientific and Educational Foundation
420 Lakeville Road
Lake Success, NY 11040
(516) 437-8100

North Carolina

Medical Review of North Carolina
1011 Schaub Drive
Booth Building
Suite 200
P.O. Box 37309
Raleigh, NC 27627
(919) 851-2955

North Dakota

North Dakota Health Care Review, Inc.
900 N. Broadway Avenue
212 Mt. Vernon Building
Minot, ND 58701
(701) 852-4231

Ohio

Peer Review Systems, Inc.
3720-J Olentangy River Boulevard
Columbus, OH 43214
(614) 451-3600

Oklahoma

Oklahoma Foundation for Peer Review
5801 Broadway Extension
Paragon Building
Suite 400
Oklahoma City, OK 73118
(405) 840-2891

Oregon

Oregon Medical Professional Review Organization (OMPRO)
1220 S.W. Morrison Avenue
Suite 300
Portland, OR 97205
(503) 243-1151

Pennsylvania

Pennsylvania Peer Review Organization
3600 Zartan Way
Harrisburg, PA 17110
(717) 652-3229

Rhode Island

Health Care Review, Inc.
The Weld Building
345 Blackstone Boulevard
Providence, RI 02906
(401) 331-6661

South Carolina

South Carolina Medical Care Foundation
P.O. Box 21667
3210 Fernandina Road
Columbia, SC 29221
(803) 798-0053

South Dakota

South Dakota FMC
608 West Avenue North
Sioux Falls, SD 57104
(605) 336-3505

Tennessee

Mid-South Foundation for Medical Care, Inc.
Penn Marc Center
6401 Poplar Avenue
Suite 400
Memphis, TN 38119
(901) 682-0381

Texas

Texas Medical Foundation
7800 Shoal Creek Boulevard
150E
Austin, TX 78757
(512) 459-3341

Utah

Utah PSRO
540 East 500 South
Suite 200
Salt Lake City, UT 84102
(801) 532-7545

Vermont

New Hampshire Foundation for Medical Care
672 Central Avenue
P.O. Box 578
Dover, NH 03820
(603) 749-1641

Virginia

Medical Society of Virginia Review Organization
1904 Byrd Avenue
Room 120
Richmond, VA 23230
(804) 289-5320

Washington

Professional Review Organization for Washington
2150 N. 107th Street
Suite 200
Seattle, WA 98133
(206) 364-9700

West Virginia

West Virginia Medical Institute, Inc.
3412 Chesterfield Avenue, SE
Charleston, WV 25304
(304) 925-0461

Wisconsin

Wisconsin Peer Review Organization
P.O. Box 1109
330 East Lakeside Street
Madison, WI 53701
(608) 257-6791

Wyoming

Montana-Wyoming FMC
P.O. Box 5117
Placer Center
21 N. Main Street
Helena, MT 59604
(406) 443-4020

Virgin Islands

Virgin Islands Medical Institute PSRO, Inc.
P.O. Box 1566, Christiansted
St. Croix, VI 00820
(809) 773-7430

Puerto Rico

Puerto Rico Foundation for Medical Care, Inc.
Mercantile Plaza Building
Suite 1520
Hato Rey, PR 00918
(809) 753-6705

B

COST-CONSCIOUS COMMUNITY CARE: RESOURCES

CAREGIVER MANUALS AND BOOKS

Coping and Caring: Living with Alzheimer's Disease (1986)
A free 24-page booklet.
AARP Fulfillment
1909 K Street, NW
Washington, DC 20049

Hand in Hand: Learning from and Caring for Older Parents (1984)
A planning guide, resource manual, and annotated bibliography.
AARP Books/Scott, Foresman and Co.
400 S. Edward Street
Mount Prospect, IL 60056

A Handbook about Care in the Home: Information on Home Health Services (1985)
A free publication of Health Advocacy Services Program Department.
American Association of Retired Persons
1909 K Street, NW
Washington, DC 20049

Information for Caregivers of the Elderly (1986)
A resource manual and instructor's manual.
Edited by S. Bane and S. Halpert.

Center on Aging Studies
University of Missouri, Kansas City
2200 Holmes Street
Kansas City, MO 64108
(816) 276-1751 or (816) 276-1747

The Loss of Self: A Family Resource for the Care of Alzheimer's Disease and Related Disorders (1986)
By Donna Cohen and Carl Eisdorfer
W.W. Norton Co.
500 Fifth Avenue
New York, NY 10110

Care Sharing Instructional Manual (1984)
Ebenezer Center for Aging
Minnesota Department of Human Services
Minneapolis, MN 55407
(612) 297-1216

Homemaker-Home Health Aide Services in Support of High-Tech Patients and Their Families (1987)
Foundation for Hospice and Home Care
519 C Street, NE
Stanton Park
Washington, DC 20002

Home Health Care: A Complete Guide for Patients and Their Families (1986)
By Jo Ann Friedman
W. W. Norton Co.
500 Fifth Avenue
New York, NY 10110

Meeting the Challenge of Disability or Chronic Illness: A Family Guide (1986)
By Lori Goldfarg et al.
Paul H. Brookes Publishing Co.
P.O. Box 10624
Baltimore, MD 21285-0624

Helping You Care: Skills Building for Home Care of the Chronically Ill Adult (1986)
Good Samaritan Hospital and Medical Center
Oregon Trail Chapter of the American Red Cross
Portland, OR

Taking Care: Supporting Older People and Their Families (1986)
By Nancy Hooyman and Wendy Lustbader

The Free Press
866 Third Avenue
New York, NY 10022

Caregiving: Helping an Aging Loved One (1985)
By Jo Horne
AARP Books/Scott, Foresman and Co.
400 S. Edward Street
Mount Prospect, IL 60056

An Approach to Training Hospice Volunteers (1981)
Beginning a Hospice (1982)
Project H.O.P.E.: A Summary (1982)
Hospice of Santa Barbara County, Inc.
330 East Carrilo Street
Santa Barbara, CA 93101

The 36 Hour Day: A Family Guide to Caring for Persons with Alzheimer's Disease, Related Dementing Illnesses and Memory Loss in Later Life (1981)
By Nancy Mace and Peter Rabins
Johns Hopkins University Press
Baltimore, MD

Gatekeeper Training Package
A video and manual to train public contact employees to identify and refer vulnerable older persons to local aging or health agencies.
National Association of State Units on Aging
233 K Street, NW
Suite 304
Washington, DC 20006
(202) 785-0707

Parent Care: Resources to Assist Family Caregivers
By Lynn Osterkamp
University of Kansas Gerontology Center
Lawrence, KS 66045
(913) 864-4130

Elder Abuse and Neglect: Causes, Diagnosis, and Intervention Strategies (1986)
By Mary Quinn and Susan Tomita
Springer Publishing
536 Broadway
New York, NY 10012

As Parents Grow Older: A Manual for Program Replication (1981)
By Alida Silverman et al.
Institute of Gerontology
University of Michigan
Ann Arbor, MI 48109

Family Seminars for Caregiving: Helping Families Help (1984)
A technical assistance manual.
Edited by Rhonda Montgomery
Pacific Northwest Long Term Care Center
Institute on Aging
University of Washington
Seattle, WA

CAREGIVER ORGANIZATIONS

As Parents Grow Older
Institute of Gerontology
University of Michigan
Ann Arbor, MI 48109

Children of Aging Parents
2761 Trenton Road
Levittown, PA 19056
(215) 547-1070

National Council on the Aging
Family Caregivers of the Aging Program
600 Maryland Avenue, SW
West Wing 100
Washington, DC 20024
(202) 479-1200

National Support Center for Families of the Aging
P.O. Box 245
Swarthmore, PA 19081
(215) 544-5933

Natural Support Program
Community Service Society
105 E. 22nd Street
New York, NY 10010

COMMUNITY VOLUNTEER PUBLICATIONS AND ORGANIZATIONS

AARP Volunteer Talent Bank
1909 K Street, NW
Washington, DC 20049

American Association of Retired Persons members, as well as nonmembers who are age 50 and over and want to volunteer, can register with the talent bank. Computerized matching will place volunteers in positions that are compatible with their interests, skills, and geographical location.

To Serve, Not to Be Served, a guide for older volunteers (1986)
American Association of Retired Persons
1909 K Street, NW
Washington, DC 20049

A free guide for improving one's chances of having a successful volunteering experience.

Older Volunteers, A Valuable Resource (1986)
American Association of Retired Persons
Program Resources Department
1909 K Street NW
Washington, DC 20049

A free guide for public and private agencies and organizations exploring the opportunity to develop volunteer programs.

Stimulating the Development of Older Volunteer Programs (1983)
By Linda Beaver and Lorraine Lidoff
National Council on the Aging
600 Maryland Avenue, SW
West Wing 100
Washington, DC 20024

A guide for establishing volunteer programs in areas, especially rural, that lack extensive service resources for older people.

Volunteer Clearinghouse
The National Center
1111 N. 19th Street
Suite 500
Arlington, VA 22209

Assists with contacting 1 of 350 centralized volunteer clearinghouses that provide a list of current voluntary opportunities and candidates for filling them.

Voluntarism in Action for the Aging (1984)
National Council on the Aging
600 Maryland Avenue, SW
West Wing 100
Washington, DC 20024
This publication encourages and assists national voluntary organizations and their affiliates with developing volunteer programs on behalf of older persons.

CONGREGATIONAL SUPPORT PUBLICATIONS AND ORGANIZATIONS

Journal of Religion and Aging
Haworth Press, Inc.
75 Griswold Street
Binghamton, NY 13904

Quarterly Papers on Religion and Aging
Oubri A. Poppele Center for Health and Welfare Studies
Saint Paul School of Theology
5123 Truman Road
Kansas City, MO 64127

Guide to Aging Programs for Synagogues
Synagogue Council of America
327 Lexington Avenue
New York, NY 10016

Gerontopics, 7 (3–4), 41–42.
Synagogues provide a variety of programs for the aged. (1986).
Newsletter on a variety of gerontology topics. This issue lists synagogues that provide programs for the aged.

Canadian Institute of Religion and Gerontology
40 St. Claire Avenue East
Suite 203
Toronto, Ontario M4T 1MG

National Interfaith Coalition on Aging, Inc.
298 South Hull Street

P.O. Box 1924
Athens, GA 30603
(404) 353-1331

Provides dissemination and advocacy for quality of life and spiritual well-being of the elderly; maintains library and promotes seminar training in gerontology.

Interreligous Liaison Office
Program Department
American Association of Retired Persons
1909 K Street, NW
Washington, DC 20049

A nonsectarian office to help churches and synagogues develop programs to meet the needs of the less fortunate elderly. Provides information brochures, films, inventory checklist of services for older persons, 10 new hymns on aging, and referral to the Widowed Persons Service.

Shepherd Center
5200 Oak Street
Kansas City, MO 64112
(816) 444-1121
Contact person: Thomas Aikens, executive director

Formed in Kansas City 15 years ago as an interfaith program for older persons. Empowerment philosophy: "No one should do for older persons what they can do for themselves." Provides numerous services to stretch the mind and spirit and promote the health of elderly (e.g., spiritual education, current event courses, arts and crafts, bereavement classes, and health and medical services). Offers no caregiver support programs as such, but strongly emphasizes home health for the frail and home repair.

The center of activity is Kansas City with one main center and 15 subcenters located in churches; but now has 50 plus centers located across the United States responding to local needs based on Kansas City model. All centers are completely run by older persons on board of directors; strong emphasis of boards and staff is advocacy around local issues.

A number of educational materials are available through the Shepherd Center (e.g., *Volunteer to Live,* a 20-minute documentary film produced by CBS on Shepherd Center programs).

ELDER CARE RESOURCES

American Association of Retired Persons
1909 K Street, NW

Washington, DC 20049
(202) 872-4700
Contact Person: Angela Heath

"Caregivers in the Workplace," an AARP women's initiative, consists of a survey to identify sources of caregiver stress in the workplace, guidelines for implementing lunchtime information fairs involving community agencies, a training package for a series of lunchtime educational sessions on caregiving and related health topics, and a training package for employee assistance counselors who may deal with employee-caregiving conflicts.

Issues for an Aging America: Employees and Eldercare
Edited by Michael Creedon
Center for the Study of Aging
University of Bridgeport
Bridgeport, CT 06601

A briefing book currently available at the National Council on Aging. This short report summarizes corporate initiatives, elder care resources for the business community, and current research efforts and provides a selected bibliography and two survey instruments on employee-caregiving.

National Association of Area Agencies on Aging
600 Maryland Avenue, SW
West Wing 208
Washington, DC 20024
(202) 484-7520
Contact person: Ed Sheehy

"Breadwinner's and Caregivers" research and demonstration project is funded by the Administration on Aging to examine the prevalence and depth of caregiving conflicts among employees. Project findings are being disseminated to area agencies on aging, along with encouragement to promote employer awareness of employee-caregiving conflicts. Approximately 700 local agencies plan, coordinate, and implement social and health support services for the 60 and over population nationwide.

WORK–SITE WELLNESS AND AGING RESOURCE ORGANIZATIONS

American Association of Fitness Directors in Business and Industry
400 6th Street, SW
Room 3030
Washington, DC 20201

Clearinghouse on Business Coalitions for Health Action
U.S. Chamber of Commerce
1615 H Street, NW
Washington, DC 20062

National Association of State Units on Aging
2033 K Street, NW
Suite 304
Washington, DC 20006
(202) 785-0707

Provides technical assistance to foster relationships between businesses and the aging network. NASUA also offers training for use of the Older Americans Act programs and products for retirement preparation. Disseminates publications such as "What Corporations Should Know about the Aging Network."

President's Council on Physical Fitness and Sports
400 6th Street, SW
Room 3030
Washington, DC 20201
(202) 272-3430

Washington Business Group on Health
229½ Pennsylvania Avenue, SE
Washington, DC 20003
(202) 547-6644

Organization houses two institutes: the Institute on Aging, Work and Health and the Institute for Worksite Wellness. Both involve businesses with state and local health and aging agencies. These institutes develop model programs for retiree organizations and provide publications, including Robert Levin's "Health Promotion for Older Persons and Retirees."

Wellness Councils of America
Wellness Council of the Midlands
Historic Library Plaza
1823 Harney Street
Suite 201
Omaha, NE 68102
(402) 444-1711

Provides information about how to organize a wellness council for a region, city, or other geographical area and how to initiate and sustain a wellness program within a business.

GERIATRIC EDUCATION CENTERS

California Geriatric Education Center
University of California at Los Angeles
Department of Medicine
Division of Geriatrics
32-144 CHS
10833 Le Conte Avenue
Los Angeles, CA 90024-1686
(213) 825-8255

Creighton Regional Geriatric Education Center
Creighton Center for Healthy Aging
42nd and Center Streets, No. 112
Omaha, NE 68105
(402) 341-1197

Dakota Plains Geriatric Education Center
University of North Dakota School of Medicine
Department of Family Medicine
221 South Fourth Street
Grand Forks, ND 58201
(701) 780-3200

Delaware Valley Geriatric Education Center
University of Pennsylvania
Center for the Study on Aging
3906 Spruce Street/H1
Philadelphia, PA 19104
(215) 898-3174

Geriatric Education Center
Department of Medicine
JHMC Box J-277
University of Florida
Gainesville, FL 32610
(904) 376-1611, ext. 5027

Geriatric Education Center
School of Public Health
144 Kron Building, 514A
University of North Carolina, Chapel Hill
Chapel Hill, NC 27514
(919) 966-5601

Geriatric Education Center
Suncoast Gerontologist Center
University of South Florida
Medical Center, Box 50
112901 N. 30th Street
Tampa, FL 33612
(813) 974-4355

Geriatric Education Center
Travelers Center on Aging
University of Connecticut
School of Medicine
263 Farmington Avenue
Farmington, CT 06032
(203) 674-3959

Geriatric Education Center
University of Alabama at Birmingham
Center on Aging
Medical Towers Building, 731
1717 11th Avenue, South
Birminghan, AL 35205
(205) 934-5619

Geriatric Education Center
Virginia Commonwealth University
Medical College of Virginia
Gerontology Department
P.O. Box 568, MCV Station
Richmond, VA 23298-0001
(804) 786-9060

Geriatric Education Center of Michigan
Department of Family Practice
B100 Clinical Center
Michigan State University
East Lansing, MI 48824
(517) 353-0770

Geriatric Education Center of Pennsylvania
Temple University Institute on Aging
University Services Building, Room 206
1601 North Broad Street
Philadelphia, PA 19122
(215) 787-6831

Geriatric Education Center
University of Puerto Rico
Sciences and Graduate School of Public Health
G.P.O. Box 5067
San Juan, PR 00936
(809) 751-2478

Great Lakes Geriatric Education Center
Chicago College of Osteopathic Medicine
5200 South Ellis Avenue
Chicago, IL 60615
(312) 947-4393

Harvard Geriatric Education Center
Division on Aging
Harvard Medical School
643 Huntington Avenue
Boston, MA 02115
(607) 732-1463

Hunter/Mt. Sinai Geriatric Education Center
Brookdale Center on Aging
Hunter College, CUNY
425 East 25th Street
New York, NY 10010
(212) 481-5142 or (212) 481-4416

Intermountain West Geriatric Education Center
University of Utah
College of Nursing
25 South Medical Drive
Salt Lake City, UT 84112
(801) 581-4064 or (801) 581-8198

Iowa Geriatric Education Center
Department of Internal Medicine
University of Iowa Hospitals
Iowa City, IA 52242
(319) 356-2727

Midwest Geriatric Education Center
Marquette University
School of Dentistry
615 North 11th Street
Milwaukee, WI 53233
(414) 224-3486

Mississippi Geriatric Education Center
Medical Alumni House
Suite 321
University of Mississippi Medical Center
2500 North State Street
Jackson, MS 39216-4505
(601) 987-4795

Missouri Geriatric Education Center
University of Missouri at Kansas City
School of Medicine
2411 Holmes
Room M5-303
Kansas City, MO 64108
(816) 474-4100

New Mexico Geriatric Education Center
Room 179 A, Nursing/Pharmacy Building
University of New Mexico
Albuquerque, NM 87131
(505) 277-0911

Northwestern Geriatric Education Center
Institute on Aging

3953 University Way, NE, JM-20
Seattle, WA 91895
(206) 545-7478

Ohio Valley/Appalachia
Regional Geriatric Education Center
University of Kentucky
20 Chandler Medical Center
Annex 1
Lexington, KY 40536-0079
(606) 233-5156

Pacific Geriatric Education Center
LAC/USC Medical Center
University of Southern California
1975 Zonal Avenue
KAM 300-C
Los Angeles, CA 90033
(213) 224-7994

Pacific Islands Geriatric Education Center
University of Hawaii Medical School
347 N. Kuakini Street
Honolulu, HI 96817
(808) 523-8461

South Texas Geriatric Education Center
University of Texas Health Sciences Center at San Antonio
Department of Dental Diagnostic Service
7703 Floyd Curl Drive
San Antonio, TX 78284-7919
(512) 691-6961

Texas Consortium of Geriatric Education Centers
Baylor College of Medicine
One Baylor Plaza
Room 134-A
Houston, TX 77030
(713) 799-4611 or (713) 799-6470

Western New York Geriatric Education Center
State University of New York at Buffalo
3435 Main Street
Beck Hall
Buffalo, NY 14214
(716) 831-3176

Western Reserve Geriatric Education Center
Department of Medicine
CWRU School of Medicine
219 Abington Road
Room W147
Cleveland, OH 44106
(216) 368-5433

Stanford Geriatric Education Center
Division of Family Medicine
Stanford University School of Medicine
703 Welch Road
Suite H-1
Stanford, CA 94305-5092
(415) 723-7063

C

COST-CONSCIOUS SELF-CARE APPROACHES: RESOURCES

HEALTH PROMOTION AND AGING BIBLIOGRAPHY

Albanese, A. A. (1980). *Nutrition for the elderly.* New York: Alan R. Liss.

American Association of Retired Persons. *Strategies for good health.* (Undated). Health Advocacy Services Program Department, 1909 K Street, NW, Washington, DC 20049.

American Association of Retired Persons. (1986). *Staying healthy after fifty: Health planner.* Washington, DC: American National Red Cross and the Trustees of Dartmouth College.

American Association of Retired Persons. (1986). *Staying healthy after fifty: Instructor's manual.* Washington, DC: American National Red Cross and the Trustees of Dartmouth College.

Arthritis: The basic facts. (1981). Atlanta: Arthritis Foundation.

Bender, R. (1976). *Be young and flexible after 30, 40, 50, 60 . . . Exercises for people in sitting occupations and for the not so young.* Avon, CT: Rueben.

Christensen, A., & Rankin D. (1979). *Easy does it yoga for older people.* San Francisco: Harper & Row.

Christensen A., & Stephenson G. (1980). *Easy does it yoga trainer's guide.* Cleveland Heights, OH: Yoga Medium Systems.

Comfort, A. (1976). *A good age.* New York: Crown.

Dartmouth Institute for Better Health, Dartmouth Medical School. (1986). *Medical and health guide for people over fifty,* Washington, DC: Scott, Foresman/American Association of Retired Persons.

Dermody, W., Saxon, V., and Scheer, E. (1986). *Successful aging program.* Clearwater, FL: Morton Plan Hospital Foundation.

deVries, A., & Hales, D. (1982). *Fitness after 50.* New York: Charles Scribners' Sons.

Dychtwald, K. (1986). *Wellness and health promotion for the elderly.* Rockville, MD: Aspen.

Etten, M. J., Hall, D. & Traynor, C. (1983). *Wealth of health: An exercise program for older adults.* Tampa: University of South Florida Suncoast Gerontology Center.

Fallcreek, S., & Mettler, M. (1982). *A healthy old age: A sourcebook for health promotion with older adults.* Seattle: University of Washington, School of Social Work, Center for Social Welfare Research.

Fallcreek, S., & Stam, S. B. (1982). *The Wallingford Wellness Project: An innovative health promotion program with older adults.* Seattle: University of Washington, School of Social Work, Center for Social Welfare Research.

Feldman, E. B. (Ed.). (1983). *Nutrition in the middle and later years.* Boston: John Wright, PSG.

Frankel, L. J., & Richard, B. B. (1980). *Be alive as long as you live.* New York: Lippincott & Crowell.

Franks, P., Lee, P., & Fullerton, J. (1983). *Lifetime fitness and exercise for older people.* San Francisco: University of California, Aging Health Policy Center.

Harris, R., Frankel, J., & Harris, S. (Eds). (1977). *Guide to fitness after fifty.* New York: Plenum.

Jamieson, (1982). *Exercises for the elderly.* New York: Alan R. Liss.

Jenkins, S. (1983). *Mental health and aging: A guide to training and program development.* Odessa, FL: Psychological Assessment Resources.

Keelor, R. (1980). *Pep up your life: A fitness book for seniors.* Hartford: Travelers Insurance.

Kemper, D., et al. (1985). *Pathways: A success guide for healthy life.* (1986). Boise: Healthwise.

Kemper, D., et al. (1986). *Growing wiser: The older person's guide to mental wellness.* Boise: Healthwise.

Kemper, D., et al. (1986). *Healthwise handbook: The practicum guide to mental wellness.* Boise: Healthwise.

Kemper, D., et al. (1987). *Growing younger handbook:* Boise: Healthwise.

Lorig, K., & Fries, J. (1980). *The arthritis helpbook.* Addison-Wesley.

Luce, G. G. (1979). *Your second life.* New York: Delacorte.

Mezey, M., Rauckhorts, L., & Stokes, S. (1980). *Health Assessment of the older individual.* New York: Springer.

Morgan, L. G. (1983). *The lifelong nutrition guide: How to eat for health at every age and stage of life.* Englewood Cliffs, NJ: Prentice-Hall.

National Institute on Aging. (1980). *A guide to medical self-care and self-help groups for the elderly.* (DHHS, Publication No. 80-1687). Washington, DC: U.S. Government Printing Office.

President's Council on Physical Fitness and Sports. (1975). *The fitness challenge . . . in the later years.* Washington, DC: Administration on Aging.

Skinner, B. F. (1983). *Enjoy old age: A program of self management.* New York: W. W. Norton.

Staying healthy: A bibliography of health promotion materials. (1984). Washington, DC: U.S. Department of Health and Human Services, Public Health Service, Office of Disease Prevention and Health Promotion.

Switkes, B. (1982). *Senior-cise: Exercises and dances in a chair.* Washington, DC: Senior-cise.

Warner-Reitz, A. (1981). *Healthy lifestyle for seniors: An interdisciplinary approach to healthy aging.* New York: Meals for Millions/Freedom from Hunger Foundation.

Weg, R. (1978). *Nutrition and the later years.* Los Angeles: University of Southern California.

RESOURCE CENTER ON HEALTH PROMOTION AND AGING

National Resource Center on Health Promotion and Aging
American Association of Retired Persons
1909 K Street, NW
Washington, DC 20049
(202) 728-4484
Contact person: Mary Gleason

DIRECTORY OF SELF-HELP CLEARINGHOUSES AND ASSOCIATIONS

The following is a combination of independent compilations of self-help clearinghouses and associations by the New Jersey Self-Help Clearinghouse, Saint Clare's Hospital, Community Mental Health Center, Ponoco Road, Denville, NJ 07834 and the Illinois Self-Help Center, 1600 Dodge, Suite 5-122, Evanston, IL 60202.

California

Sacramento Self-Help Clearinghouse
5370 Elvas
Suite B

Sacramento, CA 95819
(916) 456-2070

San Diego Self-Help Clearinghouse
1172 Morena Boulevard
San Diego, CA 92103
(619) 275-2344
Contact person: Ellen Murphy, director

San Francisco Self-Help Clearinghouse
Mental Health Association
2398 Pine Street
San Francisco, CA 94115
(415) 921-4401
Contact person: Sharon George, director

Self-Help and Mutual Aid Association (SHAMA)
c/o Alfred Katz, DSW
UCLA School of Public Health
405 Hilgard Avenue
Los Angeles, CA 90024
(213) 825-5516

Connecticut

Connecticut Self-Help/Mutual Support Network
Hamden Mental Health Center
19 Haven Street
New Haven, CT 06511
(203) 278-7645; in Connecticut, (800) 842-1501
Contact persons: Marvin Steinberg and Sophie Tworkowski, co-directors

Florida

Hillsborough County Self-Help Clearinghouse
Florida Mental Health Institute
13301 North 30th Street
Tampa, FL 33612
(813) 974-4672
Contact person: Michelle Kunkel, coordinator

Illinois

Self-Help Center
1600 Dodge Center
Suite S-122
Evanston, IL 60201
(312) 328-0470; in Illinois, (800)-322-MASH
Contact person: Daryl Isenberg, director

Kansas

Self-Help Network
Box 34
Wichita State University
Wichita, KS 67208
(316) 689-3170
Contact person: David Gleason, director

Massachusetts

Massachusetts Clearinghouse Mutual Support Groups
113 Skinner Hall
University of Massachusetts
Amherst, MA 01003
(413) 545-2313
Contact person: Warren Schumacher, director

Michigan

Berrien County Self-Help Clearinghouse
Riverwood Community Mental Health Center
2681 Morton Avenue
St. Joseph, MI 49085
(616) 983-0343

Michigan Self-Help Clearinghouse
Protection and Advocacy Service
109 W. Michigan Avenue
Suite 900
Lansing, MI 48933
(517) 484-7373; in Michigan, (800) 752-5858
Contact persons: Rob Hess and Charles Livingston

Minnesota

Minnesota Mutual Help Resource Center
Wilder Foundation Community Care Unit
919 Lanford Avenue
St. Paul, MN 55104
(612) 642-4060
Contact person: Thomas Duke, director

Missouri

Kansas City Association for Mental Health
1020 East 63rd Street
Kansas City, MO 64110
(816) 361-8563
Contact person: Barbara J. Manning

Nebraska

Self-Help Information Services
1601 Euclid Avenue
Lincoln, NE 68502
(402) 476-9668
Contact person: Barbara Fox, director

Geriatric Self-Help Center
Creighton Center for Healthy Aging
42nd and Center Streets
Omaha, NE 68105
(402) 341-1197
Contact person: David Haber, director

New Jersey

New Jersey Self-Help Clearinghouse
St. Clare's Hospital CHMC
Denville, NJ 07834
(201) 625-6395; in New Jersey, (800) 452-9790
Contact person: Edward J. Madara, director

New York

Brooklyn Self-Help Clearinghouse
Heights Hills Mental Health Service
30 3rd Avenue
Brooklyn, NY 11217
(212) 834-7341 or (212) 834-7322
Contact person: Carol Berkvist, director

Erie County Self-Help
1237 Delaware Avenue
Buffalo, NY 14209
(716) 886-1242

Long Island Self-Help Clearinghouse
New York Institute of Technology
Commack College Center
6350 Jericho Turnpike
Commack, NY 11725
(416) 499-8800
Contact persons: Robert Slotnick and Abe Jaeger, codirectors

New York City Self-Help Clearinghouse
City University of New York Graduate Center
Room 1225
33 West 42nd Street
New York, NY 10036
(212) 421-3133
Contact persons: Carol Eisman and Fran Dory, codirectors

New York State Self-Help Clearinghouse
Council on Children and Families
Empire State Plaza, 28th Floor
Albany, NY 12224
(518) 474-6293

Self-Help Clearinghouse
115 East Jefferson Street
Syracuse, NY 13202
(315) 474-7011

St. Lawrence County
Self-Help Clearinghouse
203 Sisson Hall
Potsdam, NY 13676
(315) 265-2422

St. Mary's Hospital
Self-Help Clearinghouse
427 Guy Park Avenue
Amsterdam, NY 12010
(518) 842-1900, ext. 328

Westchester Self-Help Clearinghouse
Westchester Community College
Academic Arts Building
75 Grasslands Road
Valhalla, NY 10595
(914) 347-3620
Contact person: Leslie Borck, director

Ohio

Mental Health Association of Summit County
251 E. Mill Street
Akron, OH 44308
(216) 762-7471

Oregon

Portland Self-Help Information Service
Regional Research Institute
Portland State University
1912 Southwest Sixth
Portland, OR 97207
(503) 222-5555
Contact person: Nancy Barron, director

Pennsylvania

Philadelphia Self-Help Clearinghouse
John F. Kennedy Community Mental Health Center
112 North Broad Street
7th Floor
Philadelphia, PA 19102
(215) 568-0860, Ext. 276
Contact person: Jared Hermalin, director

Self-Help Group Network of the Pittsburg Area
710½ South Avenue
Pittsburg, PA 15221
(412) 247-5400

Self-Help Information & Networking Exchange (SHINE)
Voluntary Action Center of Northeast Pennsylvania
200 Adams Avenue
Scranton, PA 18503
(717) 961-1234
Contact person: Arlene Hopkins, director

South Carolina

Support Network
Lexington Medical Center
2720 Sunset Boulevard
West Columbia, SC 29169
(803) 791-9227
Contact person: Becky Stone, director

Tennessee

Overlook Center
3001 Lake Brook Boulevard
Knoxville, TN 37909
(615) 588-9747

Texas

Dallas Self-Help Clearinghouse
2500 Maple Avenue
Dallas, TX 75201-1998
(214) 871-2420
Contact person: Carol Madison, director

Vermont

Vermont Self-Help Clearinghouse
c/o Parents Anonymous
P.O. Box 829

104 Main Street
Montpelier, VT 05602
(802) 229-5724; in Vermont (800) 554-5030

Washington, DC

Greater Washington Self-Help Coalition
(Washington, D.C., Northern Virginia, and Southern Maryland)
Mental Health Association of Northern Virginia
100 N. Washington Street
Suite 232
Falls Church, VA 22046
(703) 536-4100
Contact: Linda Figuerosa, coordinator

Wisconsin

Mutual Aid Self-Help Association (MASHA)
c/o Richard Biek, MD
1610 East Newport Avenue
Milwaukee, WI 53211
(414) 461-1466

National

Directory of National Self-Help/Mutual Aid Resources
American Hospital Association/Illinois Self-Help Center
840 North Lake Shore Drive
Chicago, IL 60611

National Self-Help Clearinghouse
City University of New York Graduate Center
Room 1206A
33 West 42nd Street
New York, NY 10036
(212) 840-7606
Contact persons: Frank Riessman and Alan Gartner, codirectors

Canada

Calgary: (403) 262-1117
Montreal: (514) 484-7406, (514) 731-8059, or (514) 392-4359
Ottawa: (613) 728-1865
Saskatchewan: (306) 652-7817
Toronto: (416) 487-4512, (416) 789-7951, (416) 863-0505, or (416) 978-3270
Victoria: (604) 721-8036
Winnipeg: (204) 589-5500, or (204) 633-5955
Initiative, national newsletter: (613) 728-1865

NATIONAL ASSOCIATIONS WITH SELF-HELP GROUP ACTIVITIES

Alzheimer's Disease and Related Disorders Association
70 East Lake Street
Chicago, IL 60601
(800) 621-1370 or (312) 853-3000

American Cancer Society
Reach to Recovery
90 Park Avenue
New York, NY 10016
(212) 599-8200

American Diabetes Association
P.O. Box 25757
1660 Duke Street
Alexandria, VA 22313
(703) 549-1500

American Heart Association
Mended Hearts/Stroke Clubs
7320 Greenville Avenue
Dallas, TX 75231
(214) 750-5300

American Lung Association
1740 Broadway
New York, NY 10019
(212) 315-8700

American Parkinson Disease Association
116 John Street
Suite 417
New York, NY 10038
(800) 223-2732 or (212) 732-9550

Amyotrophic Lateral Sclerosis Association
15300 Ventura Boulevard
Suite 315
Sherman, CA 91403
(818) 990-2151

Arthritis Foundation
3400 Peachtree Road
Atlanta, GA 30326
(404) 266-0795

Compassionate Friends (for bereaved parents)
P.O. Box 1347
Oak Brook, IL 60521

Huntington's Disease Foundation of America
250 W. 57th Street
Suite 2016
New York, NY 10107
(212) 757-0443

Make Today Count
514 Tama Building
Burlington, IA 52601
(319) 753-6521

Mended Hearts, Inc. (heart surgery aftermath)
7320 Greenville Avenue
Dallas, TX 75231

National Council on Alcoholism
12 W. 21st Street
New York, NY 10010
(212) 206-6770

National Head Injury Foundation
P.O. Box 567
Framingham, MA 01701
(617) 879-7473

National Self-Help Clearinghouse
City University of New York
33 West 42nd Street
New York, NY 10036
(305) 576-6666

National Multiple Sclerosis Society
205 E. 42nd Street
New York, NY 01017
(212) 986-3240

National Parkinson Foundation
1501 N.W. 9th Avenue
Miami, FL 33136
(305) 576-6666

THEOS Foundation (for the widowed)
Penn Hills Mall Office Building
Room 306
Pittsburg, PA 15235

United Ostomy Association
2001 West Beverly Boulevard
Los Angeles, CA 90057
(213) 413-5510

Widowed Persons Service
Program Department, AARP
1909 K Street, NW
Washington, DC 20049

PUBLICATIONS ON SELF-HELP GROUP FORMATION

Self-Help Groups: Perspectives and Directions (1978)
An instructional guide for developing self-help mutual aid groups.
By Elinor Bowles
New Careers Training Laboratory Center for Advanced Study in Education
City University of New York

Self-Help/Mutual Support Group Resources Catalogue
A guide to print and audio/visual materials for starting and maintaining mutual support groups.
California Self-Help Center
University of California, Los Angeles

2349 Franz Hall
405 Hilgard Avenue
Los Angeles, CA 90024

Starting a Self-Help Group for Caregivers of the Elderly (1984)
Children of Aging Parents
2761 Trenton Road
Levittown, PA 19056

Building Self-Help Groups among Older Persons: A Training Curriculum to Prepare Organizers
By Frances Jemmott Dory
New Careers Training Laboratory
Center for Advanced Study in Education
City University of New York

A Manual for the Development, Implementation and Operation of Family Support Groups for the Relatives of Functionally Disabled Elderly.
By Christopher Hayes
Center for the Study of Pre-retirement and Aging
Catholic University of America
Washington, DC 20064

Partners in Wellness—Self-Help Groups and Professionals
By Alfred Katz
California Department of Mental Health, Office of Prevention

Self-Care and Self Help Groups for the Elderly: A Directory (1984)
National Institute on Aging
U.S. Department of Health and Human Services
Washington, DC 20402

Self-Help Groups in Canada (1982)
Social Service Development and Grants Directorate
Health and Welfare Canada
7th Floor, Brooke Claxton Building
Ottawa, Ontario K1A 1B5

How to Start a Parkinson's Support Group
Parkinson's Educational Program
1800 Park Newport
Suite 302
Newport Beach, CA 92660

INDEX

For Product Safety Concerns and Information please contact our
EU representative GPSR@taylorandfrancis.com Taylor & Francis
Verlag GmbH, Kaufingerstraße 24, 80331 München, Germany